An Introduction to Clinical Endocrinology

An Introduction to Clinical Endocrinology

John A. Thomson
M.D., Ph.D., F.R.C.P. (Glasgow and London)
Consultant Endocrinologist, Glasgow Royal Infirmary and Royal Samaritan Hospital for Women, Glasgow;
Senior Lecturer in Medicine, University Department of Medicine, Royal Infirmary, Glasgow

SECOND EDITION

CHURCHILL LIVINGSTONE
EDINBURGH LONDON MELBOURNE AND NEW YORK 1981

CHURCHILL LIVINGSTONE
Medical Division of Longman Group Limited

Distributed in the United States of America by Churchill Livingstone Inc., 19 West 44th Street, New York, N.Y. 10036, and by associated companies, branches and representatives throughout the world.

First edition 1976
Second edition 1981

ISBN 0 443 02307 7

British Library Cataloguing in Publication Data
Thomson, John A
An introduction to clinical endocrinology. – 2nd ed.
1. Endocrine glands – Diseases
I. Title
616.4 RC648 80-41002

Printed in Hong Kong by
Wing Tai Cheung Printing Co Ltd

Preface to the Second Edition

In the five years since the first edition there have been many advances in endocrinology, especially in the application of hormone assays to clinical problems and also in methods of treating endocrine disease. In this advancing field, it is difficult to draw the line between being up-to-date and presenting methods of investigation and treatment which may be short-lived and are therefore inappropriate to an undergraduate textbook.

Some reviewers of the first edition have suggested an expansion of the physiological and biochemical data but this I have resisted since the work is intended to be used by the clinical student rather than the 2nd M. B. candidate. Similarly the book is not intended as a practical manual of endocrine investigations as this should not be part of undergraduate instruction and adequate information on the practical aspects of tests is readily available from our laboratory colleagues to junior doctors working in hospital. Rather it is intended that this small volume should be read as a broad introduction to this fascinating subspecialty of medicine.

In preparing this edition I am indebted to my colleagues Dr A. C. MacCuish and Dr I. T. Boyle who have read and made helpful suggestions about improving chapters 7 and 8 respectively.

New figures have been produced by Mrs Brenda Burn, medical artist in the University Department of Medicine.

I acknowledge the assistance of Mrs Sheila Baird and my son Alastair Thomson in proof correction and of Mrs Maureen Tucker for her secretarial help.

Lastly I must acknowledge my good fortune in working in a hospital where there is a harmonious relationship between many colleagues, both clinically and laboratory based, who have an interest in endocrine diseases. Our regular discussions have helped in the formulation of my opinions in relation to endocrine problems.

1981 J.A.T.

Preface to the First Edition

This book attempts to present an up-to-date review of clinical endocrinology at a level suitable for the undergraduate student. Since the emphasis is on the clinical aspects of the subject, anatomical, physiological and pathological data are only presented where clinically relevant. The routine biochemical tests used in clinical practice are described but details of specialised biochemical studies, for example those used to delineate the precise details of defects in cortisol or thyroxine biosynthesis, have been deliberately omitted.

References have been restricted to recent review papers or short monographs. If the student wishes to pursue any aspect of the subject in greater detail, these reviews will be found to be a useful source of reference to the original papers.

In preparing this book I have been fortunate in having had the help of many colleagues. In particular, Professor E. M. McGirr, Muirhead Professor of Medicine at Glasgow Royal Infirmary has read the whole manuscript and has made many suggestions for improving the content and style. Dr I. T. Boyle has helped me by reading the chapter on the parathyroid glands and metabolic bone disease. I am especially indebted to Mr James Y. Paton and Mr George D. Smith, 5th year medical students at Glasgow University, who read the book in an early draft form and suggested many improvements. Mrs Sheila Baird and Dr I. D. Hay assisted by reading the final draft and the proofs.

At the request of the publisher, the book has been written with laboratory values expressed as SI units. To help those who have not fully experienced the 'benefits' of the SI system, conversion factors are given in the text and an appendix of commonly used tests is provided at the back of the book. The conversion factors are quoted by permission from the booklet prepared for the Greater Glasgow Health Board by the West of Scotland Consultant Biochemists group. The figures in relation to steroid hormones and polypeptide hormones are respectively quoted by kind permission of my colleagues, Dr J. K. Grant, Reader in Steroid Biochemistry and Dr J. G. Ratcliffe, Consultant in Pathological Biochemistry, Royal Infirmary, Glasgow.

The figures used were prepared by Mrs Brenda Burn, Medical Artist in the University Department of Medicine.

I am especially grateful to my secretary, Mrs Madeleine Younger, for her work in typing the various stages of the manuscript.

1976 J.A.T.

Contents

1

The hypothalamus and the pituitary

ANATOMY

The pituitary gland is situated at the base of the brain in a hollow, the sella turcica, formed out of the sphenoid bone. The gland is composed of two parts: a) the anterior part, which takes its embryological origin from an upgrowth from the primitive mouth: this part coalesces in the sphenoid bone in embryological life with b) a downgrowth from the primitive neural tissue which goes to form the posterior part of the pituitary gland. This embryological difference is of great importance and explains the quite different functions of both parts of the pituitary and also their different control mechanisms. Since the posterior pituitary is derived from neural tissue, it has neural connections with the part of the brain immediately superior to it, the hypothalamus, whereas the anterior pituitary has no direct neural connection with the hypothalamus. The connection of the anterior pituitary with the brain is an indirect one through a capillary portal circulation by means of which the anterior pituitary receives most of its blood supply from blood which has already passed through the hypothalamus. The anterior and posterior lobes have distinct arterial blood supplies from the superior hypophyseal and inferior hypophyseal arteries respectively.

The sella turcica is roofed in by a tough membrane, the diaphragma sellae, through which passes the pituitary stalk, which constitutes the neural connection between the hypothalamus and the posterior pituitary, and also the vessels of the portal circulation to the anterior pituitary. The part of the brain above the pituitary from the optic chiasma to the mamillary bodies is the hypothalamus. As a result of much detailed work certain endocrine functions have been localised to different parts of the hypothalamus. The best known of these are the supra-optic and paraventricular nuclei in which it is thought the posterior pituitary hormones, vasopressin and oxytocin, are synthesised and then carried into the posterior pituitary gland down axons of the nerve fibres on a carrier protein, neurophysin.

In the hypothalamus are also synthesised various releasing factors which affect anterior pituitary function. Recent work has demonstrated that the hypothalamus and the pituitary form one closely integrated endocrine system. A model for the general control of anterior pituitary function by the hypothalamus is as shown in Figure 1.1. The hypothalamus synthesises releasing factors which

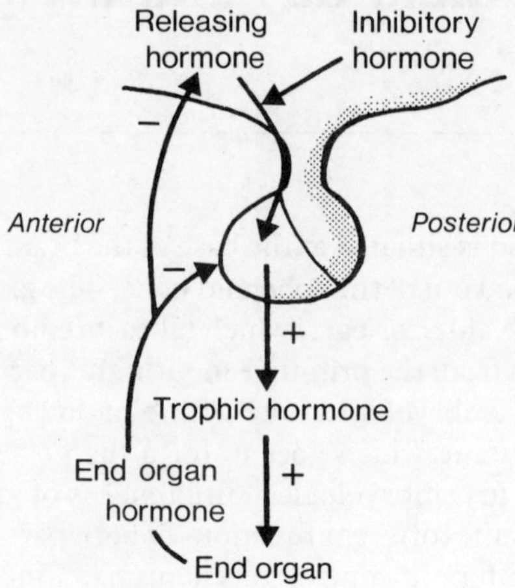

Fig. 1.1 Diagram of control of anterior pituitary function

pass down in the hypophyseal portal vessels to the anterior pituitary where they in turn stimulate the anterior pituitary to produce trophic hormones which stimulate target organs to release the end organ hormones. These end organ hormones in turn will usually effect a negative feedback control on both the pituitary and on the hypothalamus. A further control which has been shown with regard to certain releasing factors is the presence in the hypothalamus itself of a complementary inhibitory factor giving a direct local control. It has become customary to refer to those hypothalamic releasing factors which are well characterised as hormones, for example thyrotrophin releasing hormone, gonadotrophin releasing hormone, but to retain the term factor for those substances not yet fully identified.

The anterior pituitary hormones are as follows:

Hormone	*Function*
Adrenocorticotrophic hormone (ACTH)	To stimulate the adrenal cortex to produce various steroid hormones. Also stimulates adrenal growth

Growth hormone (GH)	To stimulate growth and metabolism
Prolactin	To act on the primed breast to stimulate lactation
Follicle stimulating hormone (FSH)	To stimulate follicular ripening in the ovary and spermatogenesis in the testes
Luteinising hormone, interstitial cell stimulating hormone (LH (ICSH))	To cause ovulation, to stimulate the corpus luteum of the ovary and to stimulate interstitial cell function in the testis
Thyroid stimulating hormone (TSH)	To stimulate the thyroid to produce thyroid hormones
'Melanocyte stimulating hormone' ('MSH')	To stimulate pigmentation in the skin (doubt about existence in man)

Our knowledge of the control of these various substances is still incomplete but for some the picture is becoming clearer. The best established one is the effect of thyrotrophin releasing hormone (TRH) on the stimulation of the release of TSH from the anterior pituitary. This is dealt with in the chapter on the thyroid gland. The peptide concerned is a simple tripeptide which has now been synthesised and is available for clinical use.

In relation to the control of the two gonadotrophic hormones, FSH and LH (ICSH), there is no definite evidence so far that there is a separate releasing hormone from the hypothalamus for each pituitary hormone. All the evidence at present is that a single releasing hormone, gonadotrophin releasing hormone (GnRH), will release both FSH and LH although its potency in releasing LH is much greater than in releasing FSH. GnRH has been synthesised and it is a peptide hormone which is also available for clinical use.

As regards the other releasing hormones none has been at present definitely identified as a pure chemical substance and synthesised. There are, however, fractions such as growth hormone releasing factor and ACTH releasing factor isolated from hypothalami of animals which have the action anticipated, and it is likely that such substances will be described in the future.

From the point of view of inhibitory factors, these have not been described for all hormones of the anterior pituitary and in general terms it seems to be the case that where there is a very strong negative feedback from the target organ hormone, such as the thyroid hormones, there is no local inhibitory factor present. The two best examples of inhibitory factors so far described are those in relation to prolactin and growth hormone releasing hormone.

Prolactin secretion is unusual in that it appears to be kept under normal tonic inhibitory control rather than primarily under the control of a releasing factor. This is in accord with the clinical evidence that separation of the anterior pituitary from its hypothalamic connection such as by means of stalk section results in galactorrhoea. The evidence points to the prolactin inhibiting factor being dopamine.

Growth hormone release inhibiting hormone (Somatostatin) has been isolated and synthesised. This is a potent inhibitor of growth hormone release which has been used on an experimental basis. Its development has been delayed because of its short duration of action, its need for parenteral administration and anxieties about possible effects on platelet function. However it is possible that analogues suitable for clinical use may be developed. The development of dopamine agonist drugs such as bromocriptine which are effective in lowering the elevated growth hormone levels in acromegaly is an alternative treatment which is available for oral use.

We have until now considered these releasing hormones of the hypothalamus as specific for individual pituitary hormones but this is not the case. It can readily be shown for instance that TRH in addition to releasing TSH will also release prolactin. GnRH in addition to releasing both the gonadotrophins is also capable of releasing growth hormone in certain pathological circumstances. The same lack of specificity is seen with inhibitory factors such as somatostatin, which does not only effectively inhibit growth hormone release but also inhibits the effect of TRH on release of TSH and also has an inhibitory effect on a variety of upper gastrointestinal hormones, such as insulin, gastrin and glucagon.

The problem in relating changes in the releasing or inhibitory factors to clinical endocrinology is that, in contrast to the situation with pituitary hormones, assays for the hypothalamic hormones are not available to the clinician. A further complication is that sampling from the peripheral venous blood might not reflect important changes in the hypothalamic/anterior pituitary portal system.

Clinical syndromes associated with hypothalamic disease

It is often in practice quite difficult to differentiate clinical hypothalamic disease from pituitary disease. Indeed with the new knowledge of the releasing hormones it has been realised that much of what was formerly called pituitary insufficiency is due to lack of the hypothalamic releasing hormones and not due to primary insufficiency of the pituitary itself. The converse has also been postulated, namely that apparent pituitary hyperfunction could result from primary hypersecretion of the releasing factor with subsequent pituitary overactivity.

The usual situation in which hypothalamic disease is recognised is where there is a tumour in the area of the hypothalamus causing pressure on the various nuclei. This tumour is commonly a craniopharyngioma but there are other tumours arising from the region of the optic nerve and third ventricle. In such cases features such as excessive appetite with subsequent obesity, excessive thirst or alternatively lack of the desire to drink may be seen. Excessive somnolence is also a feature. In one recent case in the author's experience there was a marked degree of electrolyte disturbance with persistently high serum sodium levels in a girl with secondary amenorrhoea. This was eventually shown to be due to a glioma arising from the region of the optic nerve.

Clinical syndromes associated with anterior pituitary hyperfunction

For each of the hormones of the anterior pituitary a clinical syndrome can be described when the hormone is present in excessive amounts.

Cushing's syndrome

So-called 'pituitary driven' Cushing's syndrome results from ACTH excess. It is fully discussed in the chapter on the adrenal.

Acromegaly and gigantism

These are the clinical syndromes resulting from sustained growth hormone excess. It is not entirely clear whether the defect is primarily in the pituitary, e.g. an autonomous growth hormone secreting tumour or whether, as has been suggested, the problem is one of primary overproduction of growth hormone releasing factor with secondary pituitary overactivity leading to adenoma formation.

Gigantism

Where growth hormone excess occurs prior to epiphyseal closure gigantism is produced whereas when the condition is found following cessation of bone growth acromegaly is produced. Gigantism is much rarer than acromegaly but most giants show well marked acromegalic features in addition to their excessive height.

In gigantism obviously the main feature clinically is excessive growth and in most cases a pituitary tumour is demonstrable radiologically. Treatment is directed at removing the growth hormone excess (see below). Obviously this requires to be done as early as possible in the course of the disease as there is no way of reversing the excessive bone growth once it has occurred.

The child with gigantism requires to be differentiated from the child who is considered by his or her parents to be abnormally tall but who has no endocrine defect. This condition has been called constitutional tall stature. It is usually found that the parents are of tall stature. It is difficult to predict the final height of the child and it may be justified in girls to give cyclical oestrogen therapy to promote early epiphyseal closure.

Acromegaly

The patient may present in a variety of ways. The term acromegaly implies increased growth of the extremities and often enlarged hands and feet are a prominent feature. In addition the patient or his friends may have noticed coarsening of facial features with increase in the soft tissues and bone overgrowth resulting in prominent supra-orbital ridges and lower jaw (prognathism). In some cases, however, the alteration in the facial features is so slow that only by comparison with photographs of some years previously is one able to notice a significant change. The voice becomes deeper due to enlargement of the larynx and thickening of the vocal cords.

Because of the increased growth of the carpal bones with consequent restriction in the carpal tunnel, patients may complain of paraesthesiae of median nerve distribution and may present because of difficulty in gripping objects. Despite what is commonly said, it is in the author's experience rather uncommon to have patients present because of headache although in most there is a radiologically demonstrable pituitary tumour present.

In addition to its growth promoting properties, growth hormone causes profound changes in fat, carbohydrate and protein metabolism. Most patients with growth hormone excess are therefore clinically hypermetabolic. They show features such as increased sweating and tachycardia and since an enlarged thyroid gland is not uncommon in acromegaly sometimes differentiation from thyrotoxicosis can be difficult. In practice most patients with acromegaly and a goitre are euthyroid. The occasional patient is indeed thyrotoxic and this is almost always due to development of one or more thyroid nodules which become autonomous. In the very exceptional patient thyrotoxicosis due to TSH excess has been described in acromegaly. One other complaint of many female acromegalic patients is that of increasing limb and body hair. This seems likely to be due to the metabolic effects of acromegaly stimulating growth of the hair follicle. Gonadotrophin insufficiency due to the pituitary tumour is common in acromegaly and is manifest by amenorrhoea in the female and impotence in the male.

Investigation. In a patient suspected of having acromegaly the diagnosis can be readily confirmed or refuted by estimation of the growth hormone during a glucose tolerance test. In the normal subject there is a reciprocal relationship between the plasma glucose and growth hormone. A normal individual will suppress his growth hormone to less than 5μU/ml when given glucose. In acromegalic patients the fasting growth hormone level is usually high and does not show suppression when glucose is administered. In some patients a paradoxical rise may even be seen in these circumstances.

In the normal individual growth hormone values vary throughout the 24 h being raised by exercise and sleep and suppressed after meals. Serial growth hormone measurements throughout the day may therefore give valuable evidence of the adequacy of growth hormone control mechanisms.

Most patients with acromegaly have a radiologically demonstrable pituitary tumour. To define the extent of the tumour especially in a suprasellar direction careful measurement of the visual fields and neuroradiological procedures such as CAT scanning and air encephalography are indicated. Various measurements of soft tissue thickening such as heel pad thickness have been described but these really add very little to the diagnosis when facilities for measuring growth hormone are available.

Treatment. When an autonomous overproduction of growth hormone has been demonstrated and X-ray examination has revealed the expected pituitary tumour, consideration must be given to treatment. In general patients with acromegaly require treatment because in its absence there is deterioration of the condition, often with increasing hypertension and death from vascular complications. In some patients however who have been undoubtedly acromegalic, the process seems to have arrested and elevated growth hormone levels are no longer found—this has been referred to as 'burnt out' acromegaly. However, this outcome is probably quite uncommon in the natural course of the disease.

Treatment aimed at lowering excessive growth hormone secretion may be either surgical, radiotherapeutic or medical.

(a) Surgical. The decision to perform a formal craniotomy in acromegaly as in other patients with pituitary tumour is made where there is a demonstrable impairment of function of the optic nerve as demonstrated by one or more visual field defects. If there is a large suprasellar extension it is easier to approach the pituitary by a formal craniotomy. In situations where there is no evidence of suprasellar extension it is preferable to tackle the pituitary from below by the transsphenoidal route. This can be done either using cryosurgical techniques, implanting radioactive sources or microsurgical techniques using the dissecting microscope.

The microsurgical approach has the advantage of allowing selective resection of small pituitary tumours and in many cases sufficient normal pituitary tissue can be left to avoid the need for permanent replacement therapy. It is not possible to obtain this degree of selectivity by 'blind' destructive techniques such as cryosurgery.

Therefore with modern surgical techniques it is possible to selectively cure early acromegaly and the aim should be to diagnose such patients as early as possible.

In larger tumours the aim of the initial operation should be to cure the acromegaly by removal of all the tumour tissue and the preservation of residual pituitary function is only of secondary importance.

(b) Radiotherapeutic. External radiotherapy used to be a frequently used treatment for acromegaly but with older techniques it was difficult to deliver an effective dose to the pituitary without running the risk of damaging other structures in the region such as the optic nerves and nerves to the extraocular muscles. Now with advances in radiotherapy, especially with proton beam therapy, there is a resurgence of interest in this method of treating acromegaly. Radioactive intrasellar implants of gold and yttrium by the transsphenoidal route have also been used with very satisfactory results.

(c) Medical treatment. Attempts have been made for some time to treat acromegaly by drug therapy. Growth hormone release inhibiting hormone (somatostatin), although theoretically attractive has not yet reached the stage of routine clinical work.

The drug most used in the medical treatment of acromegaly is the dopamine agonist bromocriptine. In normal individuals this drug raises the GH level but in acromegalic patients the paradoxical effect of lowering GH is seen. Effective control usually requires the administration of large doses (20–60 mg/day) of the drug. In these doses, apart from the usually encountered side effects of nausea and hypotension, one may encounter constipation, Raynaud's phenomenon and occasional gastrointestinal bleeding. Increasing recent interest in bromocriptine therapy has resulted from the demonstration that shrinkage of pituitary tumours, in at least a proportion of patients, may result from its use. Thus it may be used before surgery in large tumours or after operation where the tumour is not fully resectable.

It is not settled at present what the primary treatment of acromegaly should be. In the author's view, if the tumour is small and able to be selectively resected by the transsphenoidal route, it would seem logical to take this opportunity to cure the patient. In those patients not fully controlled surgically, radiotherapy or bromocriptine can be used.

Assessment of treatment

It is difficult to know what the criteria of successful treatment of acromegaly should be since there is evidence that many patients have benefited clinically from various types of treatment without a fall in growth hormone levels to normal. It can be shown in these patients that significant shrinkage of the soft tissues does occur and the patient feels better. In general, response to treatment with radiotherapy is slower than response to treatment with surgery. Indeed it is remarkable how immediate the effect of surgery is in altering soft tissue thickening both subjectively and objectively. With growth hormone values readily available there is an increasing tendency to rely on its estimation as the criterion of cure. A useful technique is to estimate GH values at intervals throughout the day and to regard cure as a mean GH value $<10\mu U/ml$.

Galactorrhoea

Galactorrhoea is the syndrome produced by excess prolactin. The name implies the production of milk from either the male breast or from the female breast not in relation to pregnancy or the puerperium.

Galactorrhoea is much commoner than is generally recognised because in clinical practice it is seldom that a patient complains spontaneously of galactorrhoea. Usually, unless it is particularly profuse, the presence of galactorrhoea is only elicited on direct questioning or as the result of examination of the breasts.

Until recently there has been controversy as to whether prolactin existed as a separate hormone in the human as it seemed to do in some animals or whether in the human, growth hormone had prolactin effects. It now seems well established by a combination of radioimmunoassay and bioassay techniques that prolactin is indeed found in the human and can be differentiated from growth hormone.

The causes of hyperprolactinaemia are outlined in Table 1.1.

Table 1.1 Causes of hyperprolactinaemia

Physiological	Neonate pregnancy lactation stress sleep
Pharmacological	Dopamine receptor blockers— Phenothiazines Metoclopramide Dopamine depleting agents— α methyldopa, reserpine Oestrogens TRH
Pathological	Hypothalamic/pituitary disease Primary hypothyroidism Renal disease Idiopathic ('functional')

Certain physiological conditions are associated with hyperprolactinaemia notably lactation, sleep and stress. It is thus important to obtain samples for prolactin estimation in as basal a state as possible. Pregnancy is associated with hyperprolactinaemia due to the effect of oestrogens acting directly on the anterior pituitary to stimulate prolactin release. A similar explanation is thought to be responsible for the transient hyperprolactinaemia of the neonate.

Drug therapy is an important cause of hyperprolactinaemia and the list includes many drugs in common use such as tranquillisers, antidepressants, oral contraceptives and antihypertensive drugs.

Amongst the pathological causes, apart from the obvious group of hypothalamic/pituitary disease, it is worth noting that renal impairment is associated with hyperprolactinaemia. Primary thyroid failure because of the negative feedback effect of increasing TRH is also associated with raised prolactin levels.

It is important to note that only about $^1/_3$ of patients with hyperprolactinaemia have clinical galactorrhoea. Thus hyperprolactinaemia is easily missed in clinical practice.

Formerly galactorrhoea had been recognised to be associated with amenorrhoea in a variety of clinical situations, for example post partum pituitary damage or in association with a pituitary tumour. Rarely, galactorrhoea may result from local trauma to the chest wall such as a thoractomy scar.

Recently however since prolactin assays have been available it has been recognised that hyperprolactinaemia associated with amenorrhoea is much more common than had been suspected—up to 20 per cent of unselected patients complaining of secondary amenorrhoea.

The current interest is in selecting from this large group of hyperprolactinaemic patients, those who are harbouring prolactin producing tumours (prolactinomas) which are too small to be radiologically apparent. Although it is only recently that such tumours have been able to be diagnosed it is clear that they are probably the most common of the pituitary tumours.

Investigation. In a patient presenting with galactorrhoea or who is found to have hyperprolactinaemia, it is important to take an adequate drug history especially with regard to use of tranquillisers or oral contraceptives and to exclude the presence of hypothyroidism before embarking on detailed studies.

The serum prolactin should be measured initially as an outpatient in as non stressed a state as possible. Normal values are 60–360mU/1. Elevated values should be confirmed by a repeat estimation to exclude those patients in whom the first sample is raised by the stress of their initial outpatient visit.

It should be noted that not every patient with galactorrhoea has a raised prolactin level.

Once drug causes and hypothyroidism have been excluded, various tests have been devised using stimulation and suppression of prolactin release. Examples of stimulation tests are those using TRH and metoclopramide and examples of suppression tests are those using bromocriptine and L-dopa. Another useful test of autonomous hyperprolactinaemia is the demonstration of loss of the normal rise in prolactin during sleep. Prolactinomas would be expected to function autonomously in these tests in contrast to the 'functional' hyperprolactinaemic states. The stimulation tests are better discriminators of pituitary autonomy since bromocriptine will suppress prolactin release from pituitary tumours as well as in 'functional' conditions.

Based on the above tests, one should be able to distinguish prolactinomas from 'functional' hyperprolactinaemia. Pituitary radiology especially by tomography should be obtained but small tumours may be present without any radiological abnormality.

Treatment. The treatment of galactorrhoea obviously depends on the cause: for instance, treatment of hypothyroidism or removal of offending drugs such as tranquillisers if these are present. A pituitary tumour, if present, may require treatment in its own right especially if it causes other endocrine effects or optic nerve compression.

With dynamic tests of prolactin secretion it has been possible to diagnose prolactinomas at a stage before radiological changes occur. Excellent results can be obtained by the methods outlined in the section on the treatment of acromegaly, namely transsphenoidal surgery, pituitary implantation and radiotherapy. In these cases, especially since often the patient desires to be pregnant, the selectivity of transsphenoidal surgery is an advantage.

Galactorrhoea was difficult to treat medically until recently when a specific prolactin inhibiting drug, bromocriptine, became available. Bromocriptine is a derivative of ergotamine and it has been shown that it will regularly inhibit elevated levels of prolactin, both in cases with and without pituitary tumours. In patients who have had long-continued hyperprolactinaemia with subsequent interference in gonadotrophin function and resultant amenorrhoea in the female and absent or low spermatogenesis in the male, the administration of this drug can result in recovery of gonadal function with ovulation in the female and spermatogenesis and resumed testosterone secretion in the male. It should be noted, however, that the induction of fertility in a female patient with a pituitary tumour puts her at risk of a sudden increase in size of the tumour during pregnancy. Some workers have therefore combined bromocriptine with radiotherapy before allowing the patient to become pregnant in the hope that this will prevent possible pituitary enlargement during pregnancy.

Another method of treating galactorrhoea medically which has been used but with less success is L-Dopa. This agent is used to diminish prolactin by increasing the prolactin inhibitory factor, dopamine.

Isosexual precosity (precocious puberty)

This is the clinical syndrome which results from premature gonadotrophin production. It is usually accepted that the onset of pubertal changes prior to the age of 9 years is abnormal. Since it is normal gonadotrophins which are being released, there is no sexual ambiguity but there is premature development of the genitalia both in the male and in the female. In the male there is development both of the penis and of the testes. In the female there is breast growth and the onset of menstruation. In both sexes pubic and axillary hair are found. In some patients a tumour in the region of the hypothalamus or the pineal gland is the cause of this premature release of gonadotrophins but in others our lack of knowledge of the precise cause of the sudden release of the gonadotrophins is merely indicative of our ignorance of the factors controlling the onset of puberty at the usual age in normal individuals.

The clinical problem in such individuals, apart from the fact that they go through puberty at an age when they are not emotionally prepared for it and obviously the females are at risk of very early pregnancy, is that the premature production of the potent anabolic hormones, testosterone and oestrogen from the gonad, as the secondary result of the gonadotrophin secretion, results in early accelerated growth but premature closure of the epiphyses and subsequent stunting. Obviously in those cases which have an associated brain tumour the prognosis is entirely dependent on whether or not the tumour is amenable to treatment.

It is important to exclude the condition of precocious puberty from that of precocious pseudopuberty, that is, where premature sexual development results from an abnormal source of androgen, such as the adrenal, or oestrogen, such as an ovarian tumour. In the male, precocious pseudopuberty will give rise to development of the penis and sex hair but not the testes which will remain small. In the female it is useful in the differential diagnosis if ovulation can be demonstrated as this would indicate true precocious puberty (that is, from a hypothalamic-pituitary mechanism of induction) in contrast to precocious pseudopuberty where ovulation is not found.

TSH excess

Theoretically, excess of TSH should result in a goitre and thyrotoxicosis. In practice thyrotoxicosis due to TSH excess has been extremely rarely described but in a few well documented patients it has been found in association with acromegaly. It must be clearly understood that the ordinary case of thyrotoxicosis is not caused by excessive production of TSH by the pituitary. In some instances thyrotoxicosis due to a TSH-like substance is found with non-endocrine tumours.

'MSH' excess

The current view is that MSH does not exist as such in the human. ACTH and MSH are derived from a larger precursor protein β-lipotrophin. ACTH itself has pigmentary properties and excessive pigmentation is seen in two clinical situations. Firstly, as part of the syndrome of Addison's disease and secondly in the condition of Nelson's syndrome, in which patients develop an invasive pituitary tumour subsequent to adrenalectomy for Cushing's syndrome. In these patients hyperpigmentation is a very striking feature and this is associated with high ACTH levels.

Clinical syndromes due to deficiency of the anterior pituitary hormones

Panhypopituitarism

Table 1.2 Causes of hypopituitarism

Idiopathic — Simmond's disease
Following obstetric haemorrhage—Sheehan's syndrome
Pituitary tumours—Chromophobe adenoma
Following treatment of pituitary tumours by surgery or radiotherapy
Granulomatous disease of the pituitary—sarcoid, TB, eosinophilic granuloma
Secondary to hypothalamic dysfunction

Usually where a patient has a lesion causing pituitary insufficiency this causes deficiency of more than one hormone. The classical clinical condition of major anterior pituitary insufficiency is called panhypopituitarism (Table 1.2) and depending on the clinical context in which it occurs a variety of other eponymous names have been attached. For instance, when the pituitary insufficiency occurs as part of severe post partum necrosis, the term Sheehan's syndrome is usually applied: when it occurs without preceding pregnancy the term Simmond's disease has been used.

Historically post partum pituitary necrosis was a very important cause of hypopituitarism in patients who survived the initial illness. Now with better obstetrical management and ready availability of resuscitative treatment it is uncommon to see new cases of Sheehan's syndrome. The syndrome resulted from the fact that the pituitary undergoes hypertrophy during pregnancy and if there was a severe haemorrhage giving a prolonged period of hypotension, there was a liability to thrombosis in the hypothalamic/hypophyseal portal system which resulted in infarction of the anterior pituitary gland.

In some patients severe hypopituitarism occurs without any obvious lesion in the pituitary or any preceding history of severe injury or illness. In at least some of these patients it can now be shown by modern techniques that the lesion is likely to be one of defective production or release of hypothalamic releasing factors rather than primary pituitary disease. In other patients severe hypopituitarism can result from a 'non-functioning' pituitary tumour although many of these so-called 'non-functioning' pituitary tumours in fact secrete excessive amounts of prolactin. Hypopituitarism can also result from granulomatous disease in the region of the pituitary especially due to tuberculous meningitis but also due to sarcoidosis and eosinophilic granuloma.

Patients with severe hypopituitarism present a typical clinical picture. Most of this can be anticipated from a knowledge of the physiology of the anterior pituitary. Usually such patients are strikingly pale due to the deficiency of ACTH. This often leads to an erroneous diagnosis of anaemia. They show features of hypothyroidism such as a dry, wrinkled skin but in contrast to hypothyroidism due to primary thyroidal failure they do not show marked thickening of the skin and subcutaneous tissue or coarsening of the hair. Indeed characteristically the head hair is of a soft, fine texture. Because of the secondary failure of release of sex steroids from the adrenal and gonads there is absent pubic and axillary hair. Because of gonadotrophin deficiency, amenorrhoea in the female and testicular atrophy in the male are regularly found. The low ACTH often will give rise to hypotension. The reason why this is not more regularly found is that aldosterone production is relatively unaffected. In those patients whose condition followed post partum pituitary necrosis, cessation of lactation due to the absence of prolactin was a regular feature. In children dwarfism is found.

The clinical diagnosis of severe hypopituitarism is therefore not difficult as the patient presents an overall unmistakable picture. Sometimes however patients with only one facet of deficient pituitary function may be seen. This is particularly found in relation to isolated deficiencies of growth hormone or the gonadotrophins.

Investigation. Investigation is directed at demonstrating lack of the various anterior pituitary and end organ hormones.

To demonstrate lack of cortisol and growth hormone an insulin tolerance test is done. Where the patient clinically is considered to show features of hypopituitarism, this must be done with great caution. A dose of 0.1 unit/kg of soluble insulin should be used as the starting dose and during the course of the test blood is taken for cortisol, sugar and growth hormone estimations. Characteristically in hypopituitarism the onset of hypoglycaemia is early and severe but there is no associated rise in the cortisol and growth hormone levels as found in the normal person. If cortisol production in response to insulin is defective it is important to confirm that the adrenal is capable of responding to exogenous ACTH before attributing the result to pituitary insufficiency (see Ch. 2).

Estimation of thyroid function by means of a serum thyroxine and triiodothyronine will confirm hypothyroidism. A low serum thyroxine will be associated with a low or absent serum TSH level in contrast to the situation in primary thyroidal failure where low circulating levels of thyroid hormone are associated with high circulating TSH values. If desired, a TSH stimulation test can be performed; it will demonstrate that the patient's thyroid is capable of responding to exogenous stimulation and by inference primary thyroidal failure is not present, thus placing the defect in the region of the pituitary or hypothalamus. A TRH test will show undetectable serum TSH levels initially with no response to administered TRH. This is in contrast to the patient with primary hypothalamic disease with secondary hypopituitarism in whom characteristically a delayed response is obtained.

Gonadal function can be assayed by measurement of the plasma oestrogen or testosterone as appropriate. In both sexes it can be shown that the circulating FSH and LH in the serum is low and in severe cases there is no response of these values to the administration of synthetic GnRH.

Treatment. In general, treatment of hypopituitarism is by replacement of the end organ hormones such as thyroxine, hydrocortisone plus oestrogen or androgen depending on the sex of the patient. Since the pituitary hormones are all polypeptide hormones their therapeutic administration remains theoretical with three exceptions. These exceptions are

1) gonadotrophin therapy to induce ovulation—this is dealt with in the chapter on the ovary.
2) growth hormone therapy in treatment of dwarfism (see below).
3) ACTH is also used as an alternative to suppressive oral steroid treatment of such conditions as asthma and ulcerative colitis occurring in endocrinologically normal patients. This is not discussed further here.

Dwarfism

When pituitary deficiency occurs before growth has been completed dwarfism will result because of the lack of growth hormone. The action of growth hormone is complex and it appears that growth hormone does not act directly on the bone to stimulate skeletal growth but instead it stimulates the production by the liver of another plasma factor, somatomedin ('sulphation factor'). It seems likely that

Table 1.3 Causes of short stature

Constitutional	low birth weight and small parental height
Chromosomal	Turner's syndrome
Environmental	nutritional, emotional deprivation
Endocrine	hypopituitarism (generalised or selective GH deficiency), hypothalamic disorders, hypothyroidism, Cushing's syndrome
Bone	achondroplasia, rickets
General Medical	malabsorption, renal disease, congenital heart disease

somatomedin acts on bone formation in conjunction with other hormones such as the sex hormones, thyroxine and adrenocortical hormones.

It must be emphasised however that growth hormone deficiency is not the major cause of failure of growth.

When presented with a child who has delayed growth, many possible conditions must be considered. First and most important is to get an accurate history of the birth weight of the child, his subsequent growth pattern and the heights of the parents and sibs. What one frequently finds is that the parental height is rather stunted or that the child is of low birth weight. Although the mechanisms involved are not fully understood, low birth weight and lack of parental height indicate that the potential for growth is not normal. One problem in assessing growth is to define what is a normal rate of

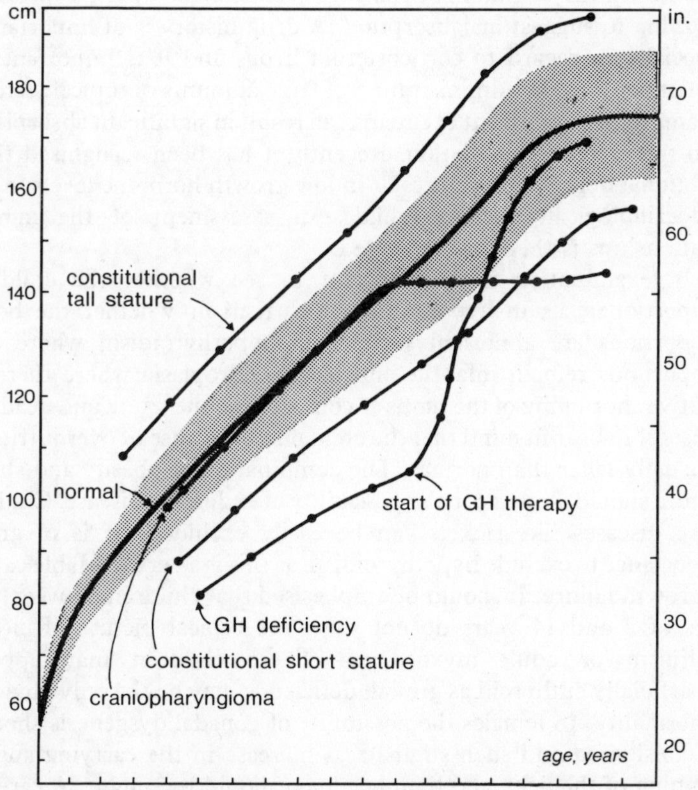

Fig. 1.2 Illustration of use of growth chart in the diagnosis of delayed and excessive growth

growth. Some form of growth chart such as the Tanner Whitehouse chart which enables the growth of an individual child to be plotted in relation to the growth of an ideal population of normal children is of great assistance in this (Fig. 1.2). Various patterns of growth may emerge. For instance one child, although small, may grow parallel to the normal growth curve. Most of these children do not have any underlying endocrine deficiency which can be demonstrated (constitutional short stature). Of much more significance is the child who has been growing normally previously but who stops growing. This would imply that some new event has taken place such as the development of a craniopharyngioma. It is also important to obtain a good history of the child's feeding habits because often on direct questioning a child who is undersized and underweight will be found to be not eating adequate amounts of food. It is also important to ask specifically for symptoms of any gastrointestinal upset, especially anything to suggest malabsorption. A drug history is of importance especially in regard to corticosteroid drugs and it is important to remember that the administration of large amounts of topical steroid creams for the treatment of eczema can result in significant absorption into the systemic circulation. Recently it has been recognised that emotional deprivation can result in low growth hormone levels in an endocrinologically normal child. An assessment of the family relationships is therefore indicated.

On examination it is important to see whether the child is proportionate as in hypopituitary dwarfism or whether the body proportions are abnormal such as in hypothyroidism where the proportions remain infantile and in achondroplasia where there is relative shortening of the limbs as compared to the trunk and head. It is useful to bear in mind that the child obese because of overnutrition is usually taller than normal. The combination of obesity and short stature should alert one to the possibility of endocrine disease. Clinical bone diseases like rickets can be easily excluded. It is of great importance to exclude hypothyroidism as this is a very treatable cause of growth failure. It should be emphasised that children between the ages of 2 and 14 years do not show the typical picture of either cretinism or adult myxoedema. These children may appear superficially euthyroid as growth deficiency may be the only obvious abnormality. In females the possibility of gonadal dysgenesis should be considered and such stigmata as increase in the carrying angle, webbing of the neck and lymphoedema should be sought. A careful assessment of the optic fundi and visual fields should be made. Dwarfism is sometimes found in the presence of serious systemic disease such as congenital heart disease or severe pulmonary disease.

This would be detected on general examination.

Investigation. The investigation of a dwarfed child is fairly obvious from the diagnostic possibilities. Tests of thyroid function such as serum thyroxine, triiodothyronine and TSH should be performed to exclude hypothyroidism. In many hypothyroid children the thyroid is present in an ectopic site and in this situation scanning of the neck may be performed although this is not required for the diagnosis of hypothyroidism. Karyotyping should be performed in any dwarfed female to exclude minor abnormalities of chromosomal constitution in patients who do not show the obvious features of gonadal dysgenesis. Tests of intestinal function should be considered, such as xylose tolerance test or faecal fat measurement and if there is any suspicion of malabsorption it is important that a jejunal biopsy should be obtained to confirm or refute the diagnosis of coeliac disease. The skull is X-rayed to demonstrate any enlargement of the pituitary fossa or any calcification above the pituitary which is frequently associated with a craniopharyngioma. Another cause of calcification above the pituitary which is relevant is healed tuberculous meningitis which may result in hypopituitarism. An X-ray of hand or other epiphyses should be performed for the assessment of bone age as typically the child with growth hormone deficiency or thyroid deficiency has a marked delay in bone development.

Growth hormone is normally released in an episodic manner especially in relation to sleep. It is also released in response to a variety of stimuli such as stress, exercise and particularly in response to a lowered level of plasma glucose. This last response is utilised clinically as a test for growth hormone release in the form of the insulin tolerance test: a normal response to adequate hypoglycaemia of less than 2 mmol/l is a rise of the serum growth hormone to greater than 20 μU/ml. A response of this magnitude effectively excludes growth hormone deficiency. A rise to less than 10 μU/ml is strongly suggestive of growth hormone deficiency especially if this is found on repeated testing. Levels between 10 and 20 μU/ml fall in the borderline category and certainly should be repeated. Although insulin is by far the most potent test for growth hormone release some paediatric consultants prefer to use, in the very young, other less dangerous provocative tests such as oral arginine, or bovril, or subcutaneous glucagon. If there is a rise of growth hormone in response to these tests to greater than 20μU/ml this is satisfactory but if a rise does not occur to these stimuli it does not mean that growth hormone deficiency has been established and this result must be confirmed by an insulin tolerance test.

An interesting group of dwarfs has been described by Laron. These children although dwarfed had high growth hormone levels and it is considered that although the growth hormone is high, there is a defect in manufacturing somatomedin, hence the poor growth.

African pygmies have also been studied. They have normal growth hormone levels and normal levels of somatomedin but it is thought that there is a true tissue refractoriness to the action of somatomedin.

After the history, clinical examination and investigation one has separated off various groups of dwarfed children and one is left with a large residue of children who fall into two main groups. Firstly there are those children who have no obvious endocrine deficiency and who have a normal bone development for their chronological age. These children would appear to be examples of constitutional short stature whose growth pattern and final height would not be influenced by treatment. Secondly there are those children who are of short stature, have delayed bone age relative to their chronological age and who usually show delayed sexual development. This latter group (who have been called constitutional delayed puberty) usually pass through puberty at a later than normal stage and grow adequately. This is in contrast to children with either isosexual precosity or those who develop sexually at a premature age because of excess androgen production from the adrenal or oestrogen from the ovary. In these children there is initial rapid growth but permanent stunting of stature due to premature epiphyseal closure.

Treatment of dwarfism. When growth hormone deficiency has been documented treatment with growth hormone should be given. In the U.K. this is obtained from the Medical Research Council and doses of 5 to 10 mg twice weekly by intramuscular injection for some years is the usual form of therapy. Normally there is rapid initial growth ('catch up' growth). In some children unfortunately growth hormone antibodies develop and growth stops. The Laron type of dwarf and the African pygmy both show an absent growth response and a poor metabolic response to GH treatment.

The treatment of other causes of dwarfism should be dealt with as they are found, for instance thyroxine therapy in hypothyroidism, gluten-free diet in coeliac disease. In certain patients, e.g. in gonadal dysgenesis, there is no treatment which is of help. It is of interest that recently it has been recognised that emotional deprivation can blunt the growth hormone response to insulin induced hypoglycaemia and this can be improved by appropriate manipulation of the environment.

Other isolated pituitary hormone deficiencies

In addition to growth hormone deficiency, isolated deficiencies of other pituitary hormones have been described. With increasing knowledge it has been realised that most of these isolated deficiencies are not primarily of pituitary hormones but are due to specific hypothalamic releasing hormone deficiencies, such as TRH deficiency causing an apparently selective TSH deficiency, GnRH deficiency resulting in apparently isolated gonadotrophin deficiency. These abnormalities are dealt with in the appropriate sections.

Pituitary tumours—general comments

Apart from pituitary tumours causing obvious endocrine disease such as eosinophil adenoma causing acromegaly or a basophil adenoma causing Cushing's syndrome, many patients present to the endocrinologist because of the finding of an enlarged pituitary fossa on X-ray. Some of these patients may also present features of lack of one or more of the pituitary hormones such as those already discussed under the heading of panhypopituitarism. In many patients, however, the finding of the expanded pituitary fossa is an accidental finding where the X-ray has been done for some other reason. In such patients it is important to assess pituitary function to make sure that there is no subclinical hormone deficiency and it is obviously important to carry out radiological investigations and ophthalmological investigations to assess the size of the pituitary tumour. It would for instance be mandatory to obtain an assessment of the visual fields in case there was any encroachment by the tumour on the optic nerves. The characteristic ophthalmological defect in pituitary tumour is a bitemporal hemianopia due to pressure on the optic chiasma catching that part of both optic nerves which crosses in the optic chiasma. It is uncommon to encounter paralysis of the 3rd, 4th and 6th cranial nerves in primary intrasellar tumours. This is however not uncommon with primary suprasellar lesions such as craniopharyngioma. Assessment of any possible suprasellar enlargement of the tumour requires such radiological techniques as tomography and CAT scanning. Cerebral angiography and pneumoencephalography are used less than formerly. Based on these various investigations a decision as to the management of the patient must be made. Where there is a significant hormone deficiency this should clearly be corrected. Where there is a sizeable suprasellar extension of the tumour, especially causing pressure on either the optic chiasma or the hypothalamus, this calls for neurosurgical treatment usually coupled with some form of radiotherapeutic treatment. Not uncommonly, however, one is faced with the patient who has no apparently demonstrable endocrine defect but who has an expanded pituitary fossa which does not seem to be causing pressure on any particular structure and in whom therefore there is no urgent indication for therapy. In such patients it has been increasingly recognised that the expanded pituitary fossa may not be as a result of a tumour and in many cases in which pneumoencephalography has been done it can be shown that the fossa can be partially filled by air. Where the person has had no preceding neurosurgical or radiotherapeutic treatment to the pituitary area this finding of a pituitary fossa which is enlarged and which can be partially or wholly filled with air on pneumoencephalography is known as the 'empty sella syndrome'. It has been suggested that such an abnormality may be commonly missed in routine clinical practice and that especially in obese patients there is an increase in the cerebrospinal fluid pressure which may cause the expanded fossa, especially if the increase in CSF pressure is coupled with a deficiency of the diaphragma sellae. Such patients with the 'empty sella syndrome' and also patients with a small pituitary tumour causing no endocrine effects do not necessarily require treatment. It is advisable to keep these patients under observation in case they develop subsequent pressure features or endocrine disease. This would be of particular importance in female patients who wished to become pregnant because of the well known tendency for the pituitary to enlarge in pregnancy.

The posterior pituitary

As already stated, the posterior pituitary is an integral part of the central nervous system. The two posterior pituitary hormones, vasopressin (antidiuretic hormone, ADH) and oxytocin are secreted in the supra-optic and paraventricular nuclei of the hypothalamus. Vasopressin is produced in response to alterations in the osmotic pressure of the perfusing plasma; oxytocin is produced in response to suckling and during parturition. These hormones pass down the axons of the nerve cells connecting the hypothalamus with the posterior pituitary bound to a carrier protein, neurophysin (Fig. 1.3). The hormones are stored in the posterior pituitary and are released as required under neural control. Vasopressin, as its name would suggest, has a pressor effect on the blood vessels but its main effect in man is that of affecting water excretion by the kidney in the collecting ducts where under its influence water is reabsorbed against an osmotic gradient. This accounts for its alternative name, antidiuretic hormone (ADH). The hormonal control of water reabsorption in this part of the renal system is very complicated. Hydrocortisone and growth hormone are two very important hormones concerned in this regulation and prolactin may also play a role.

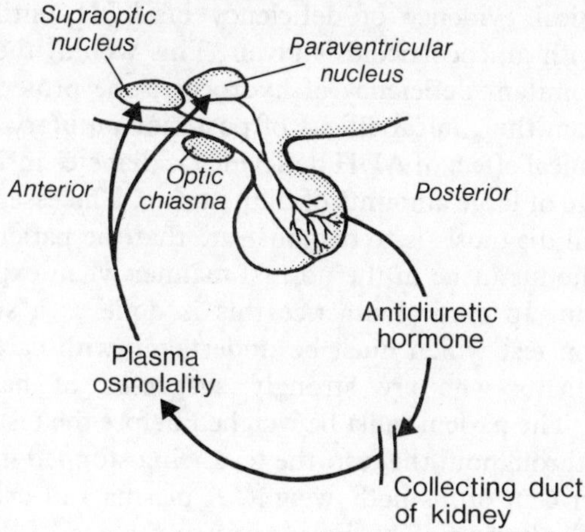

Fig. 1.3 Diagram of control of posterior pituitary function

In contrast, oxytocin whose function in animals is to assist in the initiation of labour by stimulating uterine contractions and which plays an important part in normal labour in many animals, seems not to be an essential hormone in man and there are no clinical disorders associated with its apparent deficiency. In the human female who has posterior pituitary insufficiency labour seems to take place without any undue problem and therefore no role has been definitely assigned to this hormone in human metabolism.

Deficiency of ADH

Clinical deficiency of antidiuretic hormone may occur under a variety of circumstances leading to damage of the posterior pituitary.

1. Numerically the most important is following head injury or surgical operations in the region of the pituitary and hypothalamus. It is particularly important to be aware of the possibility of posterior pituitary deficiency in these circumstances since many of these patients will be unconscious and unless a careful watch is kept on their fluid balance a serious and even fatal dehydration can result.

2. Tumours in the region of the pituitary such as intrinsic pituitary tumours and suprasellar tumours like a craniopharyngioma.

3. Inflammatory disease in the region of the pituitary, such as sarcoidosis or healed tuberculous meningitis.

4. Many of the cases are, however, not able to be ascribed to any definite cause and are labelled as idiopathic.

There is a longstanding clinical observation that patients who have complete anterior and posterior pituitary insufficiency do not show gross clinical evidence of deficiency of ADH until substitution therapy with glucocorticoid is given. This would, therefore, imply that concomitant deficiency of hydrocortisone protects the human patient from the clinical effects of posterior pituitary deficiency.

The clinical effect of ADH deficiency is diabetes insipidus, that is, the passage of large amounts of dilute urine. The essential feature in the clinical diagnosis is to demonstrate that the patient is unable to concentrate his urine in the normal manner when exposed to water deprivation. In clinical practice this is done as a standard water deprivation test which must be undertaken with care especially in those patients who are strongly suspected of having diabetes insipidus. The patient must be weighed before the test and at hourly intervals throughout the test, the test being stopped if he loses more than 5 per cent of his body weight. A plasma and urine sample are taken at the beginning of the test and at the end of the test 8 hours later. The normal response is that the urine should be able to be concentrated to greater than 650 m osm/kg by the end of the test and the plasma osmolarity should remain static around 285 m osm/kg. In a patient with diabetes insipidus the urine osmolarity will fail to reach this level but the plasma osmolarity will rise in response to dehydration. Failure of response to water deprivation should be further studied by observing the effect of ADH injection.

Differential diagnosis. The main problem in diagnosis is to differentiate diabetes insipidus from compulsive water drinking, a condition in which the affected patients are unable to stop consuming large quantities of fluid with a resulting excretion of dilute urine. Although it might seem theoretically easy to effect the separation of the two types of patient, in practice one has to take great care that these patients do not have access to water during the test. One problem which has been encountered is that some of the patients with compulsive water drinking seem eventually to develop renal tubular damage which further blurs the division between the condition of compulsive water drinking and true diabetes insipidus.

In some patients the condition of nephrogenic diabetes insipidus is encountered. This is often on a familial basis and in these patients the deficiency does not appear to be one of deficiency of the antidiuretic hormone itself but rather that the antidiuretic hormone appears to be incapable of acting in the normal way because of the abnormal response of the patient's kidneys. In such patients therefore an injection of ADH would not result in the customary concentration of the urine which is achieved in both normal subjects and patients suffering from pituitary deficiency diabetes insipidus.

Treatment. The obvious treatment of diabetes insipidus of posterior pituitary type is to replace the missing hormone. Formerly this was available in the form of pitressin tannate. However the currently available preparation is the synthetic compound DDAVP (desamino-d-argininevasopressin), 'Desmopressin'. This is a pharmacological manipulation of the vasopressin molecule in which d-arginine is substituted for the normal l-arginine in the physiological compound. This manipulation appears to make DDAVP much more resistant to breakdown in the body and therefore its action is much more prolonged. It can be used by the transnasal route for control of diabetes insipidus and is available as an intramuscular preparation.

Alternative preparations which have been used in the treatment of diabetes insipidus are:

1. Chlorpropamide. This oral agent used in the treatment of diabetes mellitus was discovered by accident to have a therapeutic effect on diabetes insipidus. It seems to act by altering the sensitivity of the renal tubules to low levels of circulating ADH. This explanation is supported by the evidence that chlorpropamide is ineffective when ADH is completely deficient. One of the side effects of using chlorpropamide in a person with normal carbohydrate tolerance is that there is a liability to attacks of hypoglycaemia if the dose used is too high. Such patients complain of attacks of weakness, often before lunch, with relief by eating. Patients with anterior pituitary deficiency are therefore particularly at risk of hypoglycaemic attacks. Another problem is that unless a careful watch is kept on the salt and water balance, undue fluid retention may be caused by chlorpropamide with resultant haemodilution.

2. Diuretics. It seems bizarre to consider diuretics in the treatment of a condition whose main clinical feature is gross and inappropriate diuresis but diuretics have a small but sometimes important part to play in the control of the condition. The mechanism of action of diuretics appears to be by depleting the intravascular compartment of salt and water, thus presenting the glomerulus with a smaller filtered load than usual. This results in a small amount of solute passing through the glomerulus and therefore a smaller amount of water arrives at the distal part of the loop of Henle to be reabsorbed or excreted. Diuretics also act in the condition of nephrogenic diabetes insipidus and they are indeed the only therapy which has any effect on this condition. It is possible on average to diminish the filtered load by the order of 50 per cent by this type of treatment.

The prognosis of diabetes insipidus depends on the cause. In those cases following head injury diabetes insipidus is often transient. In the patient who has a local lesion in the region of the pituitary, posterior pituitary deficiency is usually permanent although often clinical improvement of the diabetes insipidus is noted as increasing anterior pituitary insufficiency develops. This is of course reversed on appropriate substitution therapy for anterior pituitary insufficiency. In idiopathic diabetes insipidus the prognosis as far as life and health is good but the condition once developed seems to be permanent.

FURTHER READING

Besser G M 1974 The hypothalamus as an endocrine organ. British Medical Journal iii: 560, 613

Besser G M 1977 The hypothalamus and pituitary. Clinics in Endocrinology and Metabolism 6: 1

Brook C G D 1978 Problems of growth and development in endocrinology. In: O'Riordan J L H (ed) Recent advances in endocrinology and metabolism. Churchill Livingstone, Edinburgh, p 136–160

Chard T 1975 The posterior pituitary gland. Clinical Endocrinology 4: 89

Marshall W A 1977 Human growth and its disorders. Academic Press, Oxford

Sachs B A 1978 The brain and the endocrine system. Medical Clinics of North America 62: 2

2

The adrenal gland

APPLIED ANATOMY

The adrenal glands lie at the upper pole of each kidney. Each gland weighs approximately 4 g in the adult but in childhood the adrenals are proportionally larger. The glands have an excellent blood supply from arteries which are derived from the abdominal aorta and the phrenic and renal arteries. The arrangement of the venous drainage is of importance during surgical operations. Each gland has a central vein: the right adrenal vein is very short and drains directly into the inferior vena cava, the left adrenal vein is longer and drains into the left renal vein. Thus, it is technically much simpler to mobilise the left adrenal than to mobilise the right.

On sectioning, the adrenal gland may be seen to be composed of two distinct parts, an outer yellow cortex and an inner brown coloured medulla. The cortex is the part of the gland responsible for the synthesis of the hormones concerned with salt and water metabolism, carbohydrate regulation and certain of the sex hormones, whereas the inner part is concerned with the synthesis of adrenaline and noradrenaline. On microscopic examination the outer cortex is composed of three layers:

1. Zona glomerulosa. This outer layer in the adult is not well represented in most histological sections. It is usually recognised as small groups of cells just under the capsule. This layer is responsible for the synthesis of the important salt and water regulating hormone aldosterone.

2. Zona fasciculata. This middle layer is composed of columns of clear cells which with appropriate stains may be shown to contain lipids which are precursors of the various steroid hormones manufactured in the adrenal cortex, for example cortisol.

3. Zona reticularis. This inner layer consists of more compact cells than the zona fasciculata but there is evidence that it is composed of the same type of cell, as under ACTH stimulation the zona reticularis increases at the expense of the zona fasciculata suggesting that the latter is a precursor of the former type of cell.

The adrenal medulla is composed of argentaffin cells which are derived from the primitive neural ectoderm.

Hormones of the adrenal cortex

The adrenal cortex is capable of synthesising many different steroid hormones. These hormones are synthesised from cholesterol and all are variants of the familiar steroid ring, which is shown with the constituent carbon atoms numbered in Figure 2.1. The hormones produced (Fig. 2.2) fall into three main categories:

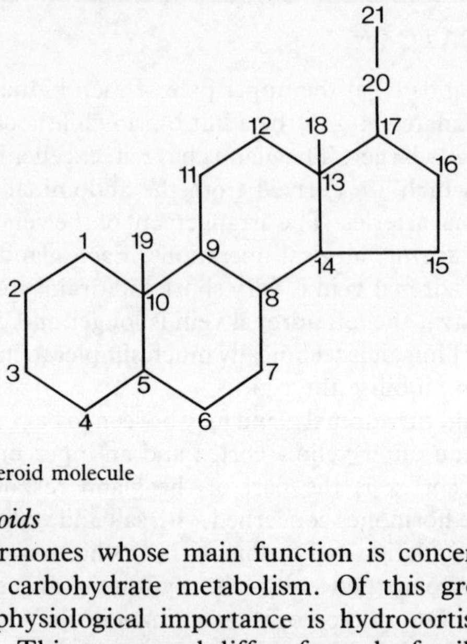

Fig. 2.1 Basic steroid molecule

1. Glucocorticoids

These are hormones whose main function is concerned with the regulation of carbohydrate metabolism. Of this group the main hormone of physiological importance is hydrocortisone (cortisol, compound F). This compound differs from the familiar pharmacological compound cortisone by having an additional hydroxyl group at position 11. When cortisone is given therapeutically it requires to be hydroxylated at this position by the liver before it is therapeutically effective.

2. Mineralocorticoids

The important compound physiologically is aldosterone. This is unusual amongst steroid compounds, in that it has an aldehyde group in position 18. It is a hormone which is extremely potent in retaining salt and water. It must be remembered, however, that the glucocorticoids such as hydrocortisone have also a salt-retaining effect and, therefore, the distinction between glucocorticoids and mineralocorticoids is to some extent artificial.

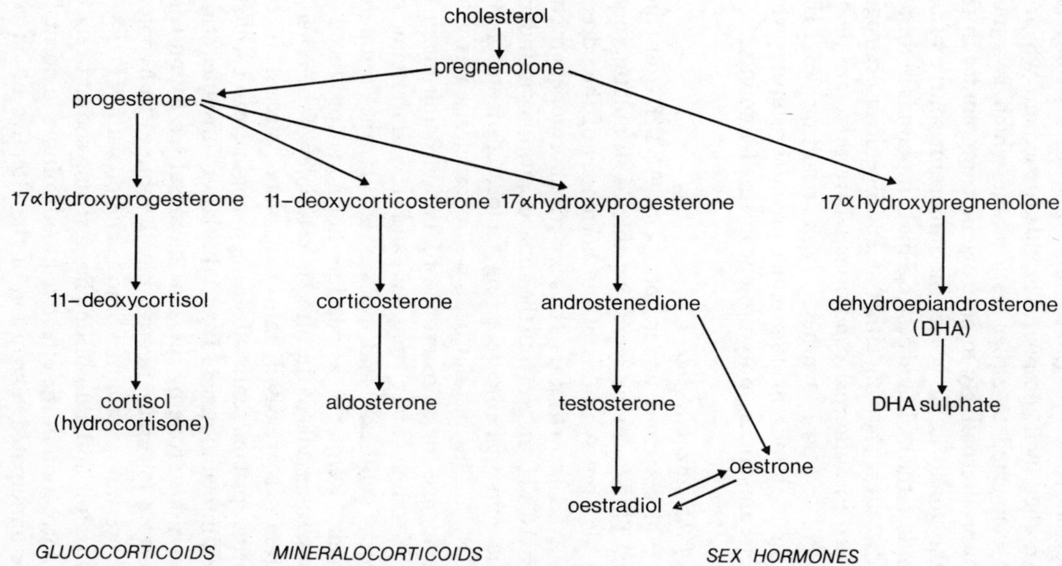

Fig. 2.2 Pathways of biosynthesis of adrenocortical hormones

3. Sex hormones

The adrenal cortex produces a variety of other hormones: some of which have androgenic effects and some of which have oestrogenic effects. Quantitatively a very important steroid hormone is dehydroepiandrosterone (DHA) and this has a weakly androgenic effect. Another such compound is androstenedione which is capable of being converted to either testosterone which is a more potent androgen or alternatively to oestrogenic compounds. In the normal person the gonad is, however, the important source of androgenic compounds in the male and oestrogenic compounds in the female, but adrenal disorders showing either an androgenic or oestrogenic effect can be seen in abnormal conditions where there are defects in the pathway of cortisol synthesis with resulting ACTH induced stimulation of the adrenal to produce precursor steroids which are, in normal circumstances, only present in small amounts.

Control of the adrenal cortex

The adrenal cortex is under control of ACTH from the anterior pituitary. This hormone seems capable of stimulating both adrenal size and also the synthesis of the hormones of the adrenal cortex, certainly as far as cortisol and the sex-active hormones are concerned.

In turn ACTH release from the anterior pituitary is under control of a specific hypothalamic releasing factor, corticotrophin releasing factor (CRF). This has not been well characterised as yet.

The evidence for aldosterone production being under control of ACTH is much more tenuous and the important control of aldosterone synthesis and release is via the renin-angiotensin mechanism. Renin is a peptide hormone produced from the juxtaglomerular cells of the afferent arterioles of the renal glomeruli. When renin is released into the blood stream it converts a polypeptide, plasma renin substrate, to angiotensin I which is in turn converted into angiotensin II and this latter substance stimulates the release of aldosterone by the zona glomerulosa. Renin is released in response to a lowered effective blood volume, to hypotension or a lowered serum sodium. Since angiotensin II is a potent vasoconstrictor and aldosterone has a strong sodium-retaining effect there is correction of the effective blood volume to normal levels. As could be anticipated, expansion of the effective blood volume and raising of the serum sodium suppress the renin-angiotensin-aldosterone mechanism.

Disorders of the adrenal cortex

Adrenocortical over-activity

1. Glucocorticoid excess

Excess production of glucocorticoid results in the appearance of the familiar condition of Cushing's syndrome. This is an uncommon disease which is usually found in young to middle-aged females. In the classical fully developed case this presents an unmistakable picture of facial plethora, central obesity which is exaggerated by loss of muscle from the limbs due to the catabolic effect of hydrocortisone, and thinning of the skin resulting in readily apparent bruising with, in addition, the appearance of broad purple striae, especially on the abdomen and over the thighs and buttocks due to the skin stretching over the increasing girth. These patients are usually hypertensive due to the sodium-retaining effect of cortisol and they may have a kyphosis due to collapse of the dorsal vertebrae. As a result of this osteoporosis with subsequent hypercalciuria, renal stone is a not uncommon complicating feature. In children with Cushing's syndrome, stunting of growth is a prominent feature. In the adult female amenorrhoea is very frequent even in those patients who do not show any other evidence of androgen excess such as hirsutism and clitoral hypertrophy. In some patients psychiatric features may be prominent ('steroid psychosis').

Although in the fully developed case the clinical diagnosis is very simple, in practice the diagnosis is often more complex especially when the patient presents with only one or two features of the disease. For instance, the patient may present primarily with osteoporosis or as a case of hypertension or of renal stone and in such cases it is important to exclude the possibility of glucocorticoid excess. Although it is always said that the main differential diagnosis is obesity due to excessive eating, in practice in most cases this does not present any great problem. In the obese patient the distribution of the obesity is quite different; striae, if present when the weight gain has been very rapid, are usually much finer, and there is not the atrophy of the skin which is seen in Cushing's syndrome. In childhood obesity due to overeating, the child is tall for his or her chronological age and not stunted as in childhood Cushing's syndrome.

It has been recognised recently that patients with chronic alcoholism can masquerade as Cushing's syndrome (alcoholic pseudo Cushings). In these patients not only may the clinical picture suggest Cushing's syndrome but the plasma and urinary steroids may be elevated. In these patients the clinical and biochemical features resolve rapidly with enforced abstinence.

Laboratory diagnosis. This falls into two stages, firstly to establish that the patient has indeed glucocorticoid excess, and secondly to differentiate between excess hormone production from primary adrenal disease (about 20 per cent of cases) and that from excessive ACTH production with secondary adrenal over-activity ('pituitary driven' Cushing's syndrome) (about 80 per cent of cases) (Fig. 2.3).

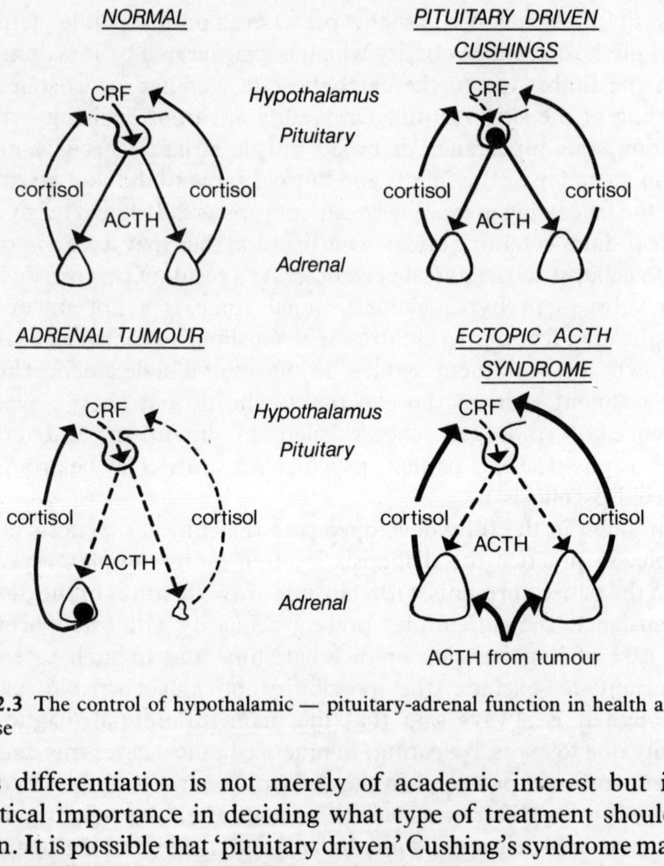

Fig. 2.3 The control of hypothalamic — pituitary-adrenal function in health and disease

This differentiation is not merely of academic interest but is of practical importance in deciding what type of treatment should be given. It is possible that 'pituitary driven' Cushing's syndrome may be due to a primary hypothalamic lesion causing excessive corticotrophin releasing factor rather than a primary disorder of the anterior pituitary. Proof of this must await the availability of assays of CRF.

The tests used to confirm glucocorticoid excess depend on the laboratory facilities available. Usually plasma 'cortisol' estimations by a fluorescent technique are available in most hospital laboratories. The general term 'cortisol' is employed in relation to the fluorescent assay as it is not entirely specific for cortisol. A common initial test is to estimate the diurnal rhythm of plasma 'cortisol'. In normal individuals there is a higher level of circulating plasma 'cortisol' in the morning, values around 700 nmol/l (conversion factor plasma 'cortisol' in nmol/l $\div 27.6 = \mu g/100$ ml), than in the evening (normal values <400 nmol/l), whereas in Cushing's syndrome the levels are not only generally higher but there is loss of this diurnal rhythm. Recent work has shown the importance of rapid bursts of adrenocortical activity at various times of the day. One isolated plasma cortisol may therefore happen to fall on a peak or a trough of such activity and give misleading results. Since the plasma cortisol is affected by stress it is very important that the estimation should be done once the patient has become accustomed to the hospital surroundings and venepuncture should be undertaken with minimal trauma. It must be remembered that certain drugs such as tetracycline and spironolactone fluoresce and therefore give falsely high results.

Cortisol in the plasma is carried mainly bound to a specific binding protein, transcortin. This protein is increased when oestrogens are administered and therefore plasma cortisol levels above the 'normal' range are found in pregnancy and in individuals on oral contraceptive drugs. It is thought that the metabolic effect is dependent on the smaller free cortisol fraction. This is normal in patients with altered transcortin values. In circumstances in which increased levels of transcortin are found a better estimation of cortisol metabolism may be obtained from tests, such as the urinary free cortisol, which are not affected by such changes in plasma cortisol transport (see below).

It is usual to estimate the adrenal response to the exogenous synthetic ACTH, tetracosactrin ('synacthen'), by doing a short synacthen test. This consists of measuring the plasma 'cortisol' before and 30 minutes after an intravenous injection of 250 mg of 'synacthen'. A normal response is an increment of plasma cortisol of > 200 nmol/l with a 30 minute value of > 550 nmol/l. One would theoretically expect that a hyperplastic adrenal would respond to ACTH in contrast to a tumour but in practice this test is not a good discriminator between tumour and hyperplasia since many adenomas do respond.

A test which has been found to be most useful in the diagnosis of glucocorticoid excess is the plasma 'cortisol' response to insulin-induced hypoglycaemia. In the normal person the plasma 'cortisol' will show an increase to values similar to that after synacthen when adequate hypoglycaemia (plasma glucose < 2 mmol/l) has been produced. The patient with glucocorticoid excess does not show any increase in the initially elevated basal values. It is obviously important that the patient should not be under any undue stress before the test as this will falsely elevate the basal 'cortisol' value and obscure any potential response.

An estimation of adrenal steroid production can be obtained from measurement of the urinary steroids. These can be measured as the 17-oxosteroids (17-ketosteroids) which are mainly products of androgen metabolism (normal values 20 to 70 μmol/24 hrs; conversion factor μmol/24 hrs ÷ 3.47 = mg/24 hrs) and are usually not raised in patients with pure glucocorticoid excess. Of more relevance are the 17-hydroxycorticosteroids which are mainly the breakdown products of cortisol (normal values 15 to 50 μmol/24 hrs; conversion factor μmol/24 hrs ÷ 3.47 = mg/24 hrs). These steroids are usually but not invariably high in Cushing's syndrome but there is a marked day to day variation in the levels and it is advisable to take several measurements before attaching too much importance to the results. The normal range of urinary steroid values varies with the age of the patient and it is important to take this into consideration. In view of the problems of obtaining reliable urine collections and the lack of specificity of estimations of the 17-oxosteroids and 17-hydroxycorticosteroids these tests are not now routinely used as a screening test in the diagnosis of Cushing's syndrome.

Theoretically a much more specific urinary test for glucocorticoid excess is measurement of the urinary free cortisol (normal value < 1000 nmol/24 hrs; conversion factor nmol/24 hrs ÷ 2.76 = μg/24 hrs). Since free cortisol but not protein bound cortisol is excreted at the glomerulus, the urinary free cortisol should reflect changes in the levels of the plasma free hormone which is thought to be the physiologically important part. This is indeed a good test for the diagnosis of Cushing's syndrome and it is one which has had an increasing place in diagnosis. A simple screening test as an outpatient is the estimation of the urinary free cortisol in an early morning urine sample, the cortisol being expressed in relation to the creatinine excretion. A normal result is < 55 μmol/mol creatinine.

These tests mentioned above, namely estimation of the plasma and urinary levels of glucocorticoids, confirm that the patient has glucocorticoid excess. They do not, however, help to define whether the glucocorticoid excess is of primary adrenal origin, e.g. adenoma or carcinoma, or due to pituitary ACTH excess. Theoretically to make this differentiation the best test would be an estimation of the plasma ACTH because this should be high in 'pituitary driven' disease but low if the adrenal is autonomously producing excess glucocorticoid. In practice, patients with glucocorticoid excess as a result of over-production of ACTH often have only modestly elevated plasma ACTH levels ranging from high-normal levels to approximately twice normal values. However, the converse finding of absent ACTH in the plasma of a patient with documented glucocorticoid excess strongly suggests the presence of an adrenal tumour (Fig. 2.3).

In the absence of facilities for ACTH estimations one has to rely on indirect tests to distinguish between adrenal and pituitary disease. The synacthen test and its shortcomings have already been mentioned. The usual test employed to distinguish between an adrenal tumour and bilateral hyperplasia is the dexamethasone suppression test which conventionally is performed in two stages. Dexamethasone is a very potent synthetic glucocorticoid which, because of the low dosage used, does not significantly interfere with steroid measurements in the blood or urine. It is given in the dosage of 2 mg per day for 2 days and then in the dosage of 8 mg per day for 2 days. The urinary 17-hydroxycorticosteroids or urinary free cortisol are measured for 2 control days preceding dexamethasone administration and for the 4 days during which it is given. A normal response is suppression of the urinary 17-hydroxycorticosteroids or urinary free cortisol during the administration of 2 mg/day in contrast to patients with Cushing's syndrome who do not suppress. Patients with 'pituitary driven' Cushing's syndrome usually show partial suppression on the 8 mg dose but patients with adrenal tumours characteristically do not. In practice the test is by no means foolproof.

An alternative approach is to use the metyrapone test. Metyrapone is a drug which blocks 11-β-hydroxylation in the adrenal cortex and therefore prevents the final stage of cortisol synthesis. In the presence of adrenal hyperplasia due to ACTH excess the effect of giving the drug is to increase greatly the precursor steroids which are measured in the urine as the 17-hydroxycorticosteroids. Where there is an adrenal tumour no such response is obtained. It is important to monitor the effect of the drug by estimating the plasma 'cortisol' to ensure that an adequate blocking effect has been achieved. If the plasma 'cortisol' has not fallen, no negative feedback response will be elicited and therefore a false negative result may be obtained. In many patients metyrapone causes severe nausea and vomiting. This can be lessened by giving the drug with milk.

X-rays of the pituitary fossa including tomography are mandatory in Cushing's syndrome but it is unusual to find a radiologically obvious pituitary tumour even when all the evidence points to excess ACTH production. Sometimes it is difficult to define the posterior clinoids because of the steroid induced osteoporosis and this may give a misleading impression to the unwary.

Where the evidence points to an adrenal tumour it is important to try to localise this to one side or the other. Formerly one had to rely on difficult and at times dangerous radiological manipulations such as aortography, perirenal air insufflation and adrenal vein catheterisation to try and show an adrenal tumour. These tests are being replaced in many centres by CAT scanning of the adrenal area and by radioisotope scanning using ^{131}I labelled cholesterol which is taken up by the adrenals. The isotope scan can be performed before and after dexamethasone administration in order to demonstrate adrenal autonomy. Since these newer tests are non invasive they can be used to demonstrate bilateral hyperplastic glands in addition to a solitary adrenal tumour. It is likely that, with improving scanning techniques, some of the present biochemical tests will become obsolete.

Treatment. Once the diagnosis has been decided it is important to embark on treatment without delay because Cushing's syndrome carries an appreciable mortality.

(a) Adrenal tumour. The simplest condition to treat is that due to an adrenal tumour. Once localisation procedures have been performed, surgical removal of the tumour should be undertaken and this would be expected to lead to cure of the condition unless the tumour was malignant. It is important to remember that once a solitary adenoma is removed, the remaining adrenal will be atrophic and steroid therapy will be required for some months until the contralateral adrenal has had the opportunity to undergo hypertrophy. It is possible to stimulate this process by giving injections of ACTH. In malignant adrenal tumours it is unusual to see a pure picture of glucocorticoid excess and therefore instead of Cushing's syndrome usually a mixed picture of glucocorticoid and androgen excess would be produced.

(b) 'Pituitary-driven' Cushing's syndrome. There is controversy in regard to the treatment of Cushing's syndrome in patients who have evidence of bilateral adrenal hyperplasia due to excessive pituitary ACTH production. One could theoretically tackle this either by dealing with the pituitary gland or with the adrenals and both approaches have their advocates.

In favour of adrenalectomy is the fact that one obtains confirmation of the diagnosis and does not miss the possibility of an undiagnosed adrenal tumour being the cause although with the scanning procedures outlined above this is less likely than formerly. By doing a total adrenalectomy one can guarantee to cure adrenocortical excess, but with the drawback of requiring permanent steroid replacement therapy as outlined under the treatment of Addison's disease. The surgical approach to the adrenal can either be through the abdomen or via a translumbar approach. Both have their advantages and disadvantages. The abdominal approach is attractive in bilateral hyperplasia as it allows both adrenals to be dealt with at one operation. Sometimes, however, the degree of abdominal obesity can create technical problems. The translumbar approach is satisfactory for adrenal tumours provided that they can be localised and are not very large.

Another problem about adrenalectomy for Cushing's syndrome is that it is followed in a proportion (about 20 per cent) of patients by marked pigmentation of the skin and the appearance of an invasive pituitary tumour which on biopsy shows the appearance of chromophobe adenoma. This sequence of events has been called Nelson's syndrome.

In favour of an attack on the pituitary itself is the fact that this deals more fundamentally with the cause of the condition, namely the excess ACTH production, but it does involve the risk of interference with other pituitary hormones and this is a consideration especially in younger women who may wish to have subsequent pregnancies. However, in many patients treated by transsphenoidal microsurgery or by pituitary implantation of yttrium, replacement hormonal therapy is not required.

In dealing with the pituitary the choice of treatment may be surgical or radiotherapeutic. In patients who have an obvious pituitary tumour, especially in those rare cases where there is any visual field defect, treatment should be by surgical hypophysectomy as outlined in the section on the treatment of pituitary tumours.

Where there is no obvious pituitary tumour successful results have been obtained by selective transsphenoidal microsurgery. The cure of Cushing's syndrome by this means would favour a primary pituitary pathology rather than a functional abnormality of the hypothalamus being the cause. Alternative approaches have been transsphenoidal implantation of radioactive pellets of yttrium or cryosurgery. For reasons already discussed these techniques are less selective than microsurgical methods.

Attempts have been made to control Cushing's syndrome with drugs, such as metyrapone, aminoglutethimide and op DDD, which have an antiadrenal effect. By themselves they have not been very effective in the long term but good results have been claimed for metyrapone in conjunction with radiotherapy, using the drug to control the clinical features of Cushing's syndrome while radiotherapy had a chance to be effective.

External radiotherapy has its advocates and there is a resurgence of interest in this type of treatment with the advent of better radiotherapeutic techniques such as proton beam therapy.

The particular technique favoured in any centre depends on the skill and experience of the people involved.

Ectopic ACTH syndrome

In some patients the clinical and biochemical picture of glucocorticoid excess can result from the secretion of an ACTH-like polypeptide from a non-endocrine tumour such as a bronchial carcinoma. This condition is discussed in detail in the chapter on endocrine effects of non-endocrine tumours.

2. *Mineralocorticoid excess*

In this condition there is an excess production of the potent salt-retaining steroid, aldosterone. Excess aldosterone production results from three separate conditions:

(a) *Primary aldosteronism (Conn's syndrome)* where the excess aldosterone production and release is due to primary adrenocortical disease. This can either be from adrenal adenoma or, more commonly recognised now, from bilateral adrenal hyperplasia. Since aldosterone is produced in excess, the plasma renin, as anticipated from physiological knowledge, is suppressed (Fig. 2.4). Such patients may present as cases of hypertension and the diagnosis should be particularly borne in mind where a hypertensive patient, who has not had any treatment such as diuretic therapy, is found to have a low serum potassium especially if combined with a moderately elevated serum sodium and a hypochloraemic alkalosis. Apart from hypertension the patient may present because of symptoms of severe potassium deficiency with weakness even verging on muscle paralysis. Characteristically there is polyuria and often glycosuria. Despite the increased body sodium the patients do not show any clinical features of excess fluid retention.

Investigation. Apart from the clinical and the electrolyte picture the specific diagnosis is made from the demonstration of a raised plasma aldosterone in the presence of an undetectable plasma renin. The response of the raised blood pressure and the correction of the electrolyte abnormalities following the use of the aldosterone antagonist, spironolactone, has been used as a diagnostic test of hyperaldosteronism. The angiotensin II antagonist, saralasin, has also been used for this purpose.

The tumour is localised as discussed under Cushing's syndrome. In Conn's syndrome the tumour is often small and may not be shown on an ultrasonic or CAT scan. Adrenal vein catheterisation may be required for biochemical localisation from the estimation of the renin in each adrenal vein and to allow adrenal venography to be performed. It is especially important to detect cases of Conn's syndrome in whom an adrenal tumour is not present as surgical treatment of these cases is not indicated. There is a great deal of interest in establishing the incidence of primary aldosteronism in hypertensive patients. Estimates have ranged as high as 20 per cent but it seems likely that the true answer is 1 per cent or less.

Treatment is either by surgical removal of an adenoma, if such can be demonstrated by localising radiological studies, or by use of an aldosterone antagonist such as spironolactone if the condition is thought to be hyperplasia.

(b) *Secondary aldosteronism.* This is a much commoner condition than primary aldosteronism and results from many situations where there is excessive fluid retention in the body, such as chronic cardiac failure, the nephrotic syndrome and especially in severe hepatic disease with ascites. In most of these states, although there is excessive fluid retention, it is thought that the fluid volume in the intravascular compartment is diminished or is sequestrated in certain areas such as the lower limbs and abdomen and this triggers the renin-angiotensin mechanism. Clearly in conditions of sodium depletion, such as after diuretic therapy, the release of renin is stimulated. In certain hypertensive patients such as those with renal artery stenosis and malignant hypertension it appears that there is secondary aldosteronism due to diminution of renal blood flow which is interpreted by the juxtaglomerular cells as a diminished effective blood volume.

In contrast to primary aldosteronism this condition is manifest by a raised aldosterone in the presence of a raised plasma renin (Fig. 2.4). Treatment is to deal with the primary disease process but the use of aldosterone antagonists is a useful adjunct to therapy.

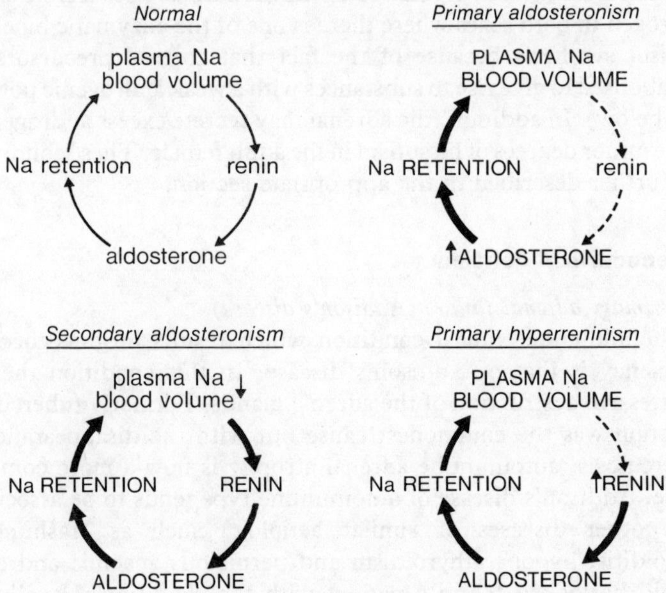

Fig. 2.4 Renin-angiotensin-aldosterone system in health and disease

(*c*) *Primary renin hypersecretion*. This is a rare entity which occurs in two circumstances:

i. where there is a tumour of the juxtaglomerular cells of the kidney resulting in an excess secretion of renin which in turn results in hyperaldosteronism. Treatment of the condition is removal of the tumour;

ii. where there is hyperplasia of the cells of the juxtaglomerular apparatus (Bartter's syndrome). These patients characteristically have marked hypokalaemia because of the renin induced hyperaldosteronism but are not hypertensive. The explanation for this discrepancy is not clear. Such patients respond to aldosterone antagonists.

3. Excess adrenal secretion of androgens and oestrogens

Since the adrenal secretes both androgens and oestrogens it is not surprising that tumours which have a virilising effect on females or a feminising effect on males have been described on rare occasions. Such tumours are nearly always malignant and rapidly lead to death of the patient. Treatment is by surgical removal where possible or if this is not feasible, to use one of the adrenal antagonists such as opDDD or aminoglutethamide. Such treatment, however, has only a temporary effect.

Apart from these malignant tumours the adrenal does secrete excess androgen in both sexes where there is one of the enzymatic blocks in cortisol synthesis because of the fact that cortisol precursors are metabolised to give rise to substances with a weak androgenic potency (see below). In addition, the adrenal may secrete excess androgens in more minor degrees of hirsutism in the adult female. These conditions are further described in the appropriate section.

Adrenocortical deficiency

1. Primary adrenal failure (Addison's disease)

In the adult the clinical condition which results in glucocorticoid deficiency is that of Addison's disease. In this condition there is progressive destruction of the adrenal glands. Formerly tuberculous infection was the commonest cause but with the disappearance of tuberculosis, autoimmune adrenal atrophy is now a more common cause. Addison's disease of autoimmune type tends to be associated with other diseases of similar aetiology such as Hashimoto's thyroiditis, hypoparathyroidism and pernicious anaemia and these should be looked for in a patient with the condition. Usually the prominent symptoms of Addison's disease are of progressive tiredness, weakness, loss of appetite, vague upper gastrointestinal symptoms and characteristically darkening of the skin. On examination pigmentation is often the first noticeable feature. Characteristically this is most marked in the exposed areas and may in some patients merely look rather like persistent suntan. In the fully developed case pigmentation is also seen on operation scars, inside the mouth, on the palmar creases and over pressure areas. Sometimes the pigmentation of the skin is patchy in distribution and associated with adjacent areas of depigmentation (vitiligo) a condition which is also frequently seen in thyrotoxicosis. In some patients, where the development of the disease has been very rapid, pigmentation may be very slight or may indeed be absent. The blood pressure is characteristically low, with systolic levels around 90 mm of mercury. Usually there are few other findings of note and unless the pigmentation is noted it is easy to dismiss such rather non-specific symptoms as functional in origin.

Diagnosis is readily made by estimating plasma cortisol which is low and the response to ACTH administration which is subnormal or absent. Usually a screening test is performed using the short 'synacthen' test, that is the intravenous injection of 250 micrograms of tetracosactrin ('synacthen') with measurement of plasma 'cortisol' before and 30 minutes after the injection. In the normal patient a rise of plasma 'cortisol' is observed. If this is not found a longer course of stimulation is given by the injection of the depot form of tetracosactrin, the dose used being 1 mg daily for 3 days following which a further 'synacthen' test is performed. If there is no rise in plasma 'cortisol' after this prolonged stimulation it can be assumed that adrenal insufficiency is present, and therapy is required. Other useful tests are X-ray of the abdomen to show adrenal calcification (in tuberculous disease), estimation of adrenal antibodies, which if present suggest autoimmune adrenal failure, and estimation of the plasma ACTH. This latter estimation would be expected to be elevated in primary adrenal failure whereas it would be low in hypopituitarism.

Other biochemical estimations of value are the blood glucose, which is often low because the action of insulin is unopposed by cortisol, accounting for part of the weakness, and the serum calcium, which is often high. This was thought to be due to the lack of glucocorticoid to counteract the alimentary absorption of calcium, but may simply be due to the diminished plasma volume.

Treatment. Most patients only require administration of hydrocortisone, the usual dosage being of the order of 20 mg in the morning and 10 mg in the evening, the equivalent dosage of cortisone acetate being 25 mg in the morning and 12.5 mg in the evening. The advantage of using hydrocortisone is that it does enable valid estimations of the plasma 'cortisol' to be made when the patient is on treatment to assess the adequacy or otherwise of the replacement dosage. Some patients require additional salt retaining steroid and this is given in the form of fludrocortisone—usually 0·05–0·1 mg per day is sufficient.

Sometimes very acute adrenocortical insufficiency can result from adrenal haemorrhage from overwhelming infections, especially meningococcal septicaemia (the Waterhouse-Friderichsen syndrome). In this condition there are usually widespread purpuric manifestations in addition to severe signs of cardiovascular collapse due to endotoxic shock and these patients require urgent large dose replacement steroids given by the intravenous route.

2. Drug-induced adrenal atrophy

Numerically a much more important group of patients with adrenal insufficiency are those resulting from the long term administration of pharmacological doses of corticosteroid drugs for such conditions as asthma or rheumatoid arthritis. Such patients have suppressed adrenal function for some months after these drugs are stopped and in some the suppression seems to be permanent. These patients are therefore at risk of developing clinical adrenal insufficiency if exposed to stress, such as surgical operations, without having additional steroid cover. It is, therefore, usual in such patients to give prophylactic treatment with a rapidly acting preparation such as intravenous hydrocortisone over the period of any operation and to follow this up with intramuscular or oral glucocorticoid for some days afterwards.

3. Secondary adrenal failure

This is due to deficiency of ACTH from hypothalamic/pituitary disease and is discussed under that heading.

4. Congenital adrenal hyperplasia

In childhood, cortisol deficiency can result from one of a series of enzymatic steps along the pathway of cortisol synthesis. This pathway is shown in diagrammatic form in Figure 2.2. Since these enzymatic defects all result in adrenal hyperplasia from excess ACTH production a general term in frequent use for this group of disorders is congenital adrenal hyperplasia.

Those defects which involve the early steps obviously give rise to very widespread deficiency of not only cortisol but many of the other hormones of the adrenal cortex such as androgens, oestrogens and mineralocorticoids. There is therefore no masculinisation of the female fetus such as is found in defects later in the pathway of cortisol synthesis where androgenic steroids are produced in excess. Indeed the external genitalia of the male fetus with a defect at the initial stages of cortisol synthesis are of female type due to the absence of androgenic steroids. Such children die shortly after birth from glucocorticoid and mineralocorticoid deficiency unless treatment is given.

Defects later along the pathway of cortisol synthesis may give rise to patients who present in early childhood with adrenal insufficiency and abnormal sexual development (precocious sexual development in the male or female pseudo-hermaphrodism — masculinisation of the external genitalia of a female fetus) due to the presence of abnormal androgen levels before full development of the external genitalia has occurred. In some defects hypertension may also be present. The hypertension is due to the secretion of cortisol precursors, such as deoxycorticosterone (DOC) and corticosterone, which is an attempted compensatory mechanism by the adrenal in response to excessive ACTH production. DOC and corticosterone are moderately potent mineralocorticoids but not effective glucocorticoids and therefore result in a salt-retaining state which leads to hypertension.

In another form there is loss of large amounts of salt in the urine and children with this salt-losing form are even more at risk of developing fatal collapse. Since this condition presents in very early childhood with mainly gastrointestinal symptoms it may be readily mistaken for some other infective or obstructive process of the gastrointestinal tract, especially when it occurs in a male infant in whom the effects of excess androgen production are less marked than in the female child. It is of the utmost importance that the diagnosis in these children is made at an early date and appropriate treatment instituted. The precise delineation of the defect is one for the specialist laboratory. The clinician must however be aware of the condition in order to make the initial steps in diagnosis and to give the appropriate therapy. This is especially so since the condition is an inherited one and therefore can be seen in other members of the family.

Treatment consists of the administration of saline, fludrocortisone and an adequate dosage of glucocorticoid to give effective circulating levels of adrenal hormones. This treatment in turn results in diminution of the adrenal size because of suppression of ACTH production and also results in suppression of the formation of precursors of cortisol which are present in excessive amounts and which, as noted above, may be androgenic. Patients who have marked degrees of virilisation may require plastic surgery later to correct ambiguity of the external genitalia. Shortness of stature is common in these patients because of either inadequate treatment resulting in premature epiphyseal closure from high androgen levels or from excessive glucocorticoid therapy exerting a catabolic effect on the bones.

It should be noted that in a few patients the defect is only partial and such patients may not present until around puberty or even as adults with mild degrees of virilisation.

5. Congenital adrenal hypoplasia

This is a rare condition in which the clinical picture of severe adrenal insufficiency is associated with hypoplastic adrenals. It too is a familial disorder, the treatment of which is with adequate steroid replacement.

Mineralocorticoid deficiency

This is almost never seen as an isolated entity because not only does aldosterone have a salt-retaining action but so do the glucocorticoid hormones which would be able to compensate. Mineralocorticoid deficiency is therefore only seen in association with severe glucocorticoid deficiency. It should be noted that most patients with Addison's disease do not under ordinary circumstances show an electrolyte defect even in the absence of treatment. Where there is an exacerbation of the condition they may well show a low sodium and a high serum potassium but this indicates a dangerous deterioration of their condition. Since aldosterone production is not primarily under control of ACTH, patients who have primary pituitary disease usually do not show such severe electrolyte problems as patients who have primary adrenal disease.

It has been suggested that in some elderly patients a primary deficiency of renin might exist with secondary hypoaldosteronism. The incidence of this has not been defined.

Deficiency of sex hormones of adrenal origin

Since in normal circumstances in either sex the adrenal only plays a minor role in the production of oestrogens or androgens there is not usually any clinical deficiency of sex hormone production attributable to adrenal disease. The ovary in the female and the testes in the male are, if normal, able to compensate for any potential deficiency which might result from adrenal disease.

The adrenal medulla

The adrenal medulla is really a specialised portion of the sympathetic nervous system. It secretes the characteristic hormones involved in the neural transmission in the sympathetic chain, namely adrenaline and noradrenaline. These hormones have their main effect on the cardiovascular system, shown by an acceleration of the pulse, a rise in blood pressure and increased cardiac output. They also cause shutting down of the blood flow in the skin vessels in order to maintain the central part of the circulation.

Catecholamine excess

The classical condition in which this is found is in phaeochromocytoma which is a tumour of the adrenal medulla. This tumour is usually simple but on rare occasions can be malignant and may occasionally be bilateral. Sometimes bilateral phaeochromocytomas are found associated with an unusual thyroid tumour, medullary carcinoma. In this condition the syndrome is often familial with an autosomal dominant pattern of inheritance.

The diagnosis of phaeochromocytoma is usually made on investigation of a patient with hypertension, especially where there is any suggestion of paroxysms of hypertension associated with systemic features such as palpitations, sweating, blanching of the skin, faintness and severe headaches. In all patients with severe hypertension an estimation of catecholamines should be performed before therapy is instituted as many of the drugs used in the treatment of hypertension interfere with the assay. The type of assay done depends on the laboratory. The most common is estimation of the urinary catecholamine metabolites (metadrenaline and normetadrenaline). Another popular screening test is estimation of the urinary vanillylmandelic acid (VMA). Sometimes plasma catecholamines can be estimated. Stimulatory tests with histamine and tyramine and suppressive tests with catecholamine antagonists such as phentolamine ('Rogitine', known as 'Regitine' in North America) have now generally been abandoned as being both misleading and dangerous.

Following the biochemical confirmation of the diagnosis the tumour must be localised and this is usually best performed by aortography since a phaeochromocytoma is a vascular tumour and is readily outlined by this technique. Alternative techniques are CAT scanning, ultrasonic scanning and adrenal vein catheterisation. On occasions even after these techniques have been used, the tumour may not be localised. This is especially so if it is in an extra-adrenal site. In this case catheterisation of the inferior vena cava to allow sampling of blood for estimation of the plasma catecholamines at various levels may aid in the localisation.

The correct treatment is surgical but this must be done after appropriate preparation of the patient. The management of the condition has been revolutionised by the advent of effective alpha and beta adrenergic blocking drugs, such as phenoxybenzamine and propranolol respectively, and these are given before and during the operation. Once the tumour has been removed there is often a marked fall in the blood pressure and intravenous noradrenaline and hydrocortisone are usually required for the first postoperative day or so.

Deficiency of catecholamines

There is no definite documented disease associated with destruction of the adrenal medulla.

Other tumours of the adrenal medulla

These are uncommon except in the neonate in whom neuroblastoma is found. This tumour is a malignant one which often spreads widely. Surgical treatment followed by radiotherapy provides the only hope of cure.

The other type of tumour found is the ganglioneuroma which is at least initially a non-malignant tumour.

In both of these tumours there may be evidence of abnormal metabolism of catecholamines and their precursor compounds but usually there are no clinically obvious endocrine effects.

FURTHER READING

Brown J J, Fraser R, Lever A F, Robertson J I S 1972 Hypertension with aldosterone excess. British Medical Journal ii: 391

Lansberg L 1977 Catecholamines. Clinics in Endocrinology and Metabolism 6: 3

Mason A S (ed) 1972 Disease of the adrenal cortex. Clinics in Endocrinology and Metabolism 1: 2

3

The thyroid gland

ANATOMY

The thyroid gland is situated in the lower anterior part of the neck. It overlies the thyroid cartilages and the upper end of the trachea, being closely attached to these structures by the pretracheal fascia, which accounts for the clinical observation that the thyroid gland moves on swallowing thus helping to differentiate it from other swellings in that part of the neck. In the adult the thyroid gland weighs approximately 25 g. It consists of a bilobed structure connected by a narrow strip of tissue, the isthmus. From the isthmus an additional portion of thyroid tissue extending upwards in approximately the mid-line of the neck may be noted, especially in certain pathological conditions. This is the pyramidal lobe of the thyroid. This upward extension reminds us of the embryology of the thyroid gland which originates from the base of the tongue and descends in the mid-line of the neck to the adult site during fetal life. The site of origin of the thyroid is marked by the foramen caecum at the junction of the anterior two-thirds and posterior one-third of the tongue. Sometimes remnants of thyroid tissue may be found along this line of descent; indeed on occasion the patient's only functioning thyroid tissue may be in such an abnormal site without any thyroid tissue present in the normal position.

The thyroid obtains its blood supply from paired superior and inferior thyroidal arteries and the venous drainage is to the internal jugular and innominate veins. The lymphatic drainage is mainly to the lateral lymph nodes of the neck.

The normal thyroid gland consists of circular follicles containing an amorphous mass of protein material, the colloid, surrounded by a rim of cuboidal epithelial cells. The follicles are in turn surrounded by connective tissue containing blood vessels and the lymphatics; the capillary vessels in particular are placed in very close juxtaposition to the basement membrane of the epithelial cells. In addition to the thyroid epithelial cell there are other cells which may be seen by special stains. These are not epithelial cells but are so-called 'C' cells or light cells. These latter cells are thought to be the cells responsible for production of the calcium-lowering hormone, calcitonin.

Formation of the thyroid hormones

The thyroid gland manufactures two main hormones concerned with control of metabolism. These hormones are thyroxine (T_4) and tri-iodothyronine (T_3). Their formation within the thyroid results from a complicated series of biochemical steps, which is outlined in Figure 3.1. An important constituent of both hormones is iodine and,

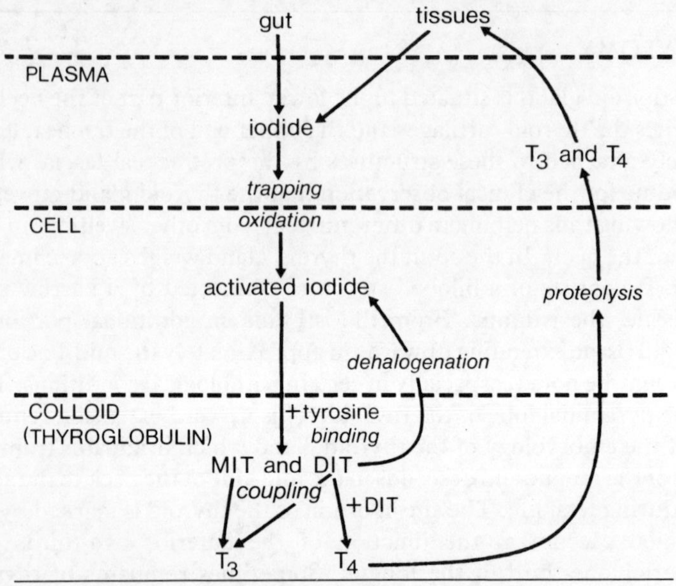

Fig. 3.1 Pathways of thyroid hormone biosynthesis

therefore, the first step consists of the accumulation by the thyroid of iodine from the plasma passing through it. The thyroid is very efficient at trapping iodine and once trapped, the iodine is very rapidly changed in the thyroid cell to an activated form of iodine, the precise nature of which is not clear. It probably results from the activity of peroxidase enzymes which are present in the thyroid. The oxidized iodine is rapidly bound to the tyrosine molecules which exist as part of the molecules of thyroglobulin. This substance is a very large glycoprotein whose initial formation occurs independently of the iodine content. The iodination of tyrosine residues produces either mono-iodotyrosine (MIT) or di-iodotyrosine (DIT) depending on the numbers of iodine atoms in each tyrosine residue. Where sufficient iodinated tyrosine residues are present these coalesce to form the hormones T_3 and T_4. It will, therefore, be noted that the thyroid hormones are not formed as free entities but as part of the thyroglobulin molecule. When thyroglobulin is broken down by proteolytic enzymes, the thyroid hormones T_3 and T_4 are released as required into the plasma in the capillaries round the thyroid follicles and are transported into the general circulation.

In the plasma the thyroid hormones travel mainly bound to specific binding proteins, the most important of which is thyroxine binding globulin (TBG). Another thyroxine binding protein, thyroxine-binding pre-albumin (TBPA) has also been described. T_3, like T_4, is bound to proteins in the plasma but is much less firmly bound and is therefore relatively much more available for controlling the metabolic state. The protein bound hormones are in equilibrium with a smaller free fraction which is thought to be the important fraction in controlling metabolism. Unfortunately free T_3 and free T_4 are present in such small amounts that their measurement is not at present a routine test. Although thyroxine is contained in the thyroid gland in a ratio of 9:1 as compared to T_3 there is now considerable evidence that at least half the metabolic effect of the hormones depends on T_3. The weaker binding affinity of T_3 compared to T_4 makes it more readily available to the tissues. T_3 has also greater biological potency per molecule than T_4. There is now evidence that much of the circulating T_3 comes not from thyroidal secretion but from the deiodination of T_4 to T_3 in the peripheral blood. Circulating T_4 can either be deiodinated to the more active T_3 or to the virtually inactive reverse T_3 (r T_3). Thus there is an additional control of thyroid metabolic effect in the peripheral circulation. There is still controversy as to whether T_4 itself is metabolically active or whether transformation to T_3 is an essential preliminary step.

The thyroid hormones have a multiplicity of effects, the most obvious being the alteration of the metabolic state of the body, but there also are profound effects on fat, carbohydrate and protein metabolism. It is impossible in terms of current knowledge to say which one of these effects is the prime one.

Control of the thyroid gland

The thyroid gland is under control of the pituitary by means of the pituitary hormone, thyroid stimulating hormone (TSH). This is produced from specific beta cells in the anterior pituitary. TSH is in its turn under the control of the hypothalamic releasing hormone, thyrotrophin releasing hormone (TRH). There is evidence that at both pituitary and hypothalamic level there is a negative feed-back control by means of the circulating thyroid hormone levels so that a raised level of circulating thyroid hormone will shut off release of the TSH and TRH respectively.

Tests of thyroid function

These tests can be grouped into five main classes.

1. Those which estimate the circulating thyroid hormones.
2. Estimation of serum TSH.
3. TRH test.
4. Those which examine the function of the thyroid gland itself.
5. Those which measure the peripheral action of the thyroid hormones.

Many tests of thyroid function have been described, all of which have their particular applications and drawbacks and it is important that the appropriate test should be selected to elucidate the particular clinical problem under study.

1. Tests measuring the circulating thyroid hormones

Tests falling within this category are the estimation of the protein bound iodine (PBI), serum total thyroxine (serum total T_4), serum total tri-iodothyronine (serum total T_3) and the thyroid hormone uptake test (THUT). As previously mentioned measurement of the free hormone levels is not at present a practical routine test.

The protein bound iodine was for a considerable time the standard test of thyroid function of this group. The introduction of this test was a significant advance because it provided the first test of thyroid function giving a quantitative estimate of the circulating thyroid hormone values as estimated from their iodine content as opposed to indirect tests using radioactive iodine. It is a simple and cheap test especially when automated techniques of estimation are used but it has been superseded in clinical practice because:

1. there are problems of interfering substances containing iodine (see section on thyroid uptake);
2. it is interfered with by pathological conditions or drugs altering the levels of the circulating TBG and other binding proteins;
3. we now have available tests which measure the serum total T_4 and total T_3 directly and not indirectly by means of their iodine content, as in the case of the PBI.

The serum total T_4 can be measured by means of a radioimmunoassay or by a competitive protein binding system. Normal values are of the order of 60 to 150 nmol/l (conversion factor, serum T_4 in nmol/l $\times 0{\cdot}0777$ = serum T_4 in μg/100 ml). This test is not affected by iodine administration but is affected by alterations in TBG content (see below).

The serum total T_3 value is estimated by a radioimmunoassay procedure. The normal range is 1–3 nmol/l (conversion factor, serum total T_3 in nmol/l × 0·651 = serum T_3 in ng/ml).

Thyroid hormone uptake test (THUT)

This is a measure of the number of unoccupied T_4 and T_3 binding sites on the patient's serum proteins. It is estimated by means of a T_3 resin uptake test. It is important that this test is clearly distinguished from estimation of the serum total T_3 value. The THUT is a very useful test in clinical practice, not because it is a particularly good test of thyroid function but because by this simple test one can infer changes in the circulating TBG levels. This is important in conditions such as the administration of oestrogen, especially in the form of oral contraceptives, or during pregnancy where TBG is increased, falsely high serum total T_4 and serum total T_3 values being obtained. Conversely in cases where the TBG value is lowered, falsely low serum total T_4 and serum total T_3 results are found.

The principle of the thyroid hormone uptake test is illustrated in Figure 3.2. An *in vitro* system is set up in which there is a competitive

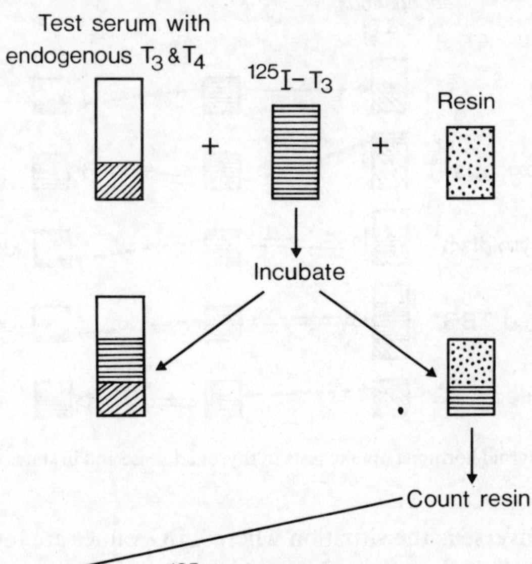

$$T_3 \text{ resin uptake} = \frac{{}^{125}I\text{–}T_3 \text{ counts on resin}}{\text{Initial } {}^{125}I\text{–}T_3 \text{ counts}} \times 100$$

Fig. 3.2 Principle of thyroid hormone uptake test

equilibrium between the patient's serum proteins, which contain TBG, added radioactive T_3, and an inert acceptor of T_3 which is usually a resin sponge or a loose resin. In thyrotoxicosis where most of the serum binding sites are occupied by the endogenous thyroid hormones, there is an increased resin uptake of the added radioactive T_3. The converse is found in hypothyroidism where because of the large number of unoccupied binding sites on the serum proteins there is very little uptake of the added radioactive T_3 on the resin sponge.

This situation is, however, complicated in the presence of altered TBG values. The common situation to encounter in clinical practice is increased TBG values from the effect of oestrogen, either as a result of pregnancy or of the administration of the oral contraceptive pill. In this situation there is an increase in TBG, which causes a compensatory increase in thyroid hormones, as shown by the estimation of the serum total T_4 or serum total T_3 values. However, because of the increased number of binding sites available, there is a greater uptake, in the THUT, of the added radioactive T_3 by the patient's serum and therefore a falsely low THUT is obtained (Fig. 3.3).

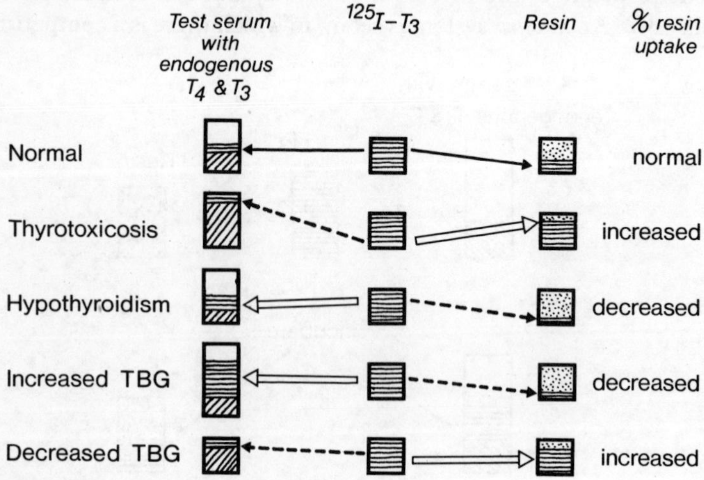

Fig. 3.3 Thyroid hormone uptake tests in thyroid disease and in states of altered TBG binding

The converse is the situation where TBG values are lowered. This usually occurs when there is gross hypoproteinaemia such as in the nephrotic syndrome or where certain drugs such as androgens, which lower the TBG level, are used. Anticonvulsants of the phenytoin group or analgesics such as salicylates which are able to bind to thyroxine binding sites also give an apparently lowered TBG level. In these conditions because there are fewer unsaturated TBG sites available there is less uptake of the added labelled T_3 on to the TBG of the patient's serum and, therefore, a greater uptake of the labelled T_3 on to the resin. This results in a falsely elevated THUT.

It will be noted we therefore have a situation that where there is an increased TBG binding capacity there is a falsely high serum total thyroxine and a falsely low THUT. In cases where there is diminished TBG binding capacity there is a falsely low serum total thyroxine and a falsely high THUT. The THUT may therefore be used to correct the value of the serum thyroxine by taking account of these alterations in TBG capacity. This correction is made by dividing the serum T_4 value by the THUT expressed as a percentage of a normal pooled serum. This is known as the free thyroxine index (FT_4I).

2. Estimation of the serum TSH

Since the thyroid gland is controlled by means of the pituitary TSH secretion, it would appear likely on theoretical grounds that estimation of TSH would be a useful test of thyroid function. This is so where the question of hypothyroidism arises. In this condition where there is disease affecting the thyroid gland itself, such as autoimmune atrophy of the thyroid, post-irradiation or post-thyroidectomy, the failing thyroid is stimulated by an increased level of serum TSH which, therefore, provides a sensitive test for the detection of mild degrees of hypothyroidism. Where thyroidal failure is as a result of pituitary failure there should theoretically be no detectable TSH present. Estimation of the serum TSH is not a useful test in diagnosis of possible thyrotoxicosis. In this condition one would anticipate that the serum TSH would be lower than normal. While this may be true, current assay procedures do not have sufficient sensitivity to reliably detect values which are less than normal. Normal values for the serum TSH vary from laboratory to laboratory but are of the order of 0 to 8 mU/l.

TRH test

Since TSH in turn is controlled by the TRH secretion from the hypothalamus the availability of synthetic TRH has opened up the possibility of other tests of thyroid function. When TRH is administered to a normal person the serum TSH rises rapidly with a peak value of around 12 mU/l occurring around 20 minutes and a fall-off to values around 8 mU/l occurring over a period of one hour. Where the initial TSH is already raised as in primary thyroidal failure, there is an exaggerated response of the serum TSH to the administration of TRH. Usually, however, there is very little place in clinical practice for TRH tests in the diagnosis of mild degrees of hypothyroidism since the simple estimation of the serum TSH provides the necessary information. In patients who have a hypothalamic lesion in whom there has been a lack of stimulation by TRH over a long time, the TSH response in the serum to a test dose of TRH is characteristically delayed with higher values being obtained at 60 minutes than at 20 minutes.

The main usefulness of the TRH test is in the diagnosis of possible hyperthyroidism. In this condition, since the patient's pituitary and hypothalamus are exposed to constant high levels of circulating thyroid hormones, one would anticipate that there is suppression of TSH and TRH release by the negative feed-back mechanism. When a test dose of TRH is administered to such patients there is characteristically no rise in plasma TSH.

4. Tests of thyroid gland function

These are tests which measure some aspect of the thyroid gland function and in the 1950s and 60s were the most important tests of thyroid function available. They have now, largely, been superseded by tests involving the measurement of the circulating thyroid hormones. Tests of the thyroid gland involve the use of radioactive isotopes of iodine. The simplest test of this group is measurement of the uptake by the thyroid of radioactive iodine. This can be estimated at various times after administration of a test dose of the isotope. The most widely used measurement is a 24 hour thyroid uptake; the normal range of the measurement varies slightly from area to area but is of the order of 15 to 40 per cent at 24 hours. Other uptake times can be used and other common ones are early times such as 4 hours, or late times such as 48 hours, after administration of the test dose. Early uptakes have certain advantages in the diagnosis of thyrotoxicosis whereas late uptakes are more helpful in the diagnosis of possible hypothyroidism. The test was often completed by measuring the turnover of radioactive iodine within the thyroid by means of estimating the 48 hour protein bound ^{131}I. This gives an estimate of the proportion of the dose administered which is turned into thyroid hormone over the 48 hour period of study. This is increased in thyrotoxicosis when values of greater than 0·4 per cent of dose per litre of plasma are found, values below this being found in normal subjects and in patients with hypothyroidism.

Two main fallacies affect radio-iodine studies. One is the administration of inorganic iodine usually in the form of cough mixtures and various radio-opaque dyes. These interfere with the iodine uptake by a mass action effect. The other main problem is patients who have a small functioning thyroid reserve. In such patients the intra-thyroidal turnover of iodine is accelerated and, therefore, a falsely high 48 hour $PB^{131}I$ is obtained due to the unduly rapid transit of iodine within the thyroid. This occurs in patients who have had a thyroidectomy, in those who have had radio-iodine therapy, in patients who have a solitary hyperfunctioning nodule and in patients with progressive destructive lesions of the thyroid such as Hashimoto's thyroiditis.

Although radio-iodine studies have a high diagnostic accuracy they are not so much used as formerly because of the fact that they are time-consuming both for the patient and staff and they require administration of radioactive isotopes of iodine. For these reasons when the question to be answered is simply to decide whether the patient is thyrotoxic, euthyroid or hypothyroid, *in vitro* tests of thyroid function are preferred.

Recently, especially in North America, increasing numbers of cases of thyrotoxicosis associated with subclinical thyroiditis have been recognised. In these patients there is the paradoxical condition of increased thyroid hormone release resulting in thyrotoxicosis which is however associated with a suppressed thyroid uptake of ^{131}I. The importance of recognising these cases is that destructive therapy with radio-iodine or surgery should be avoided in their management.

The main indication now for doing radio-iodine studies of the thyroid is where a thyroid scan is also desired. This applies mainly where a patient has an apparently solitary nodule in the thyroid, when a scan is done to assess whether the nodule is normally functioning thyroid tissue or whether it shows impaired function which might suggest a thyroid neoplasm. Thyroid scanning in these situations is dealt with under the subject of the solitary thyroid nodule.

The other group of patients in whom radio-iodine studies are performed as a routine are patients with thyrotoxicosis who are to be treated with radio-iodine. In these patients the thyroid uptake is used to assess the therapeutic dose.

5. Tests based on peripheral action of the thyroid hormones

The best known test in this group is the basal metabolic rate. This is a classical test of thyroid function which has fallen into disfavour because it is cumbersome to perform. It is now no longer used in routine practice.

Estimation of the Achilles tendon relaxation time results from the well established clinical observation that in patients with hypothyroidism the tendon reflexes are delayed, particularly in the relaxation phase. A commercial apparatus is available which allows for the measurement of this relaxation phase by means of a mechanical tendon hammer attached to a photometric recording device. This test is used in some centres but is not generally favoured. Its diagnostic usefulness is limited. The method is indirect. Nowadays direct estimation of the thyroid hormones and TSH is preferred.

Diseases of the thyroid gland

Thyrotoxicosis

Thyrotoxicosis may occur in several well recognised forms:

1. A diffusely enlarged over-active thyroid associated with exophthalmos (Graves' disease).
2. Thyrotoxicosis due to a single hyperfunctioning thyroid nodule (Plummer's disease).
3. Neonatal thyrotoxicosis.

Graves' disease

Aetiology. This is one of the two major forms of thyrotoxicosis. Characteristically it affects women during the reproductive years, the incidence in men being only about one-sixth of that in women. The cause of this condition remains controversial. It was originally suggested that the pituitary might be over-active and stimulate the thyroid gland by means of TSH. This theory can be discounted except in *very* exceptional instances where a pituitary tumour releases high levels of TSH. In 1956 the description of long-acting thyroid stimulator (LATS) which is an abnormal 7S gamma globulin present in the serum of some patients with the disease, led to the suggestion that LATS was the cause of the thyroid stimulation. This theory has been progressively eroded to the point at which it is no longer tenable as the main cause of thyrotoxicosis. More recently there has been a shift of interest to another abnormal stimulatory substance referred to as LATS protector (LATSP). The current view is that there is a group of substances referred to collectively as thyroid stimulating immunoglobulins (TSI) which are present in the serum of patients with Graves' disease. The techniques of identifying and measuring these compounds are not yet developed to the level of identifying the precise protein fraction involved and there is controversy about the correct nomenclature. It is hoped that this will be clarified in the near future.

From the clinical standpoint stress is a postulated cause for thyroid over-activity and there is no doubt that stress is often seen in patients coming to a thyroid clinic. There is equally well no doubt that many patients are severely stressed who do not develop thyroid disease and a striking example of this was the marked fall in the incidence of thyrotoxicosis in occupied Europe during the Second World War. The only exception to this epidemiological evidence was in Denmark where there was an increased incidence.

Clinical features. The patient with Graves' disease presents, in the fully developed state, an unmistakable clinical picture which may be recognised by an experienced observer at a glance. The clinical features may be considered under four groups:

1. The peripheral manifestations of thyroid hormone excess.
2. Changes in the thyroid gland.
3. Changes in the eyes.
4. Other features.

1. The peripheral effects of thyroid hormone excess are largely mediated via catecholamines. This explains the tachycardia, the increased sweating, tremor, nervousness. This group of manifestations can all be controlled to a large extent by the administration of an effective beta adrenergic blocking drug such as propranolol. In some patients, especially in the older age groups, the cardiac effects may predominate. Arrythmias, especially atrial fibrillation, but also supraventricular tachycardia, are common. Such patients may present with angina due to rapid heart action or with intractable cardiac failure. This condition has been referred to as 'masked' thyrotoxicosis and it is very important to remember the possibility of thyrotoxicosis as a cause of high output cardiac failure especially in cases who seem to be resistant to the effects of digoxin.

2. The thyroid gland in Graves' disease is characteristically symmetrically enlarged. It is usually well defined with a well marked pyramidal lobe. It is often about 60 to 80 g, that is about 3 to 4 times normal size. Typically the thyroid gland in Graves' disease is diffusely enlarged but with longstanding disease the gland may be multinodular especially if there is a history of preceding non-toxic goitre. The consistency is rather rubbery. In severe cases there is a well marked thrill on palpation over the thyroid and an audible bruit on auscultation over the gland. A thyroid bruit is systolic in time and must be clearly differentiated from venous hums in the neck which may be readily heard in an anxious patient. The latter can be easily differentiated by showing that they are obliterated by venous occlusion above the region of the thyroid.

3. The eye features of thyrotoxicosis vary in different patients and may indeed be completely absent. The simplest feature is retraction of the upper lid due to the excessive adrenergic effect on the levator

palpebrae superioris. This effect is also shown on getting the patient to follow the examiner's finger from looking in an upward direction to looking down, in which case the upper lid will lag behind the iris resulting in the exposure of white sclera between the two structures. This sign is therefore referred to as 'lid lag'. The term exophthalmos implies actual protrusion of the eyes which can be measured if one so desires by an exophthalmometer. In most severely affected cases infiltration and oedema of the conjunctiva (chemosis) are seen and in particularly severely affected cases there is involvement of the extraocular muscles which results in paresis of one or more of the muscles. This paresis gives rise to diplopia which the patient usually first notices on attempting to look upwards. Various extraocular muscles may be involved culminating in occasional cases in inability to move the eyes in any direction (complete ophthalmoplegia). Even more rarely the pressure in the orbital contents may increase to such a degree that papilloedema or optic atrophy may result. These severe degrees of eye involvement in thyrotoxicosis are referred to as malignant exophthalmos. It should be emphasised that not every patient with Graves' disease develops significant eye involvement and in those patients with exophthalmos the condition is not usually progressive. Exophthalmos may be predominantly unilateral. In patients with unilateral exophthalmos in the absence of obvious thyrotoxicosis the possibility of intraorbital tumours should be remembered. However, it is not uncommon in thyrotoxic patients to see unilateral exophthalmos. Conversely, some patients may present with the eye features of Graves' disease without being thyrotoxic. This is referred to as ophthalmic Graves' disease. About half such patients eventually become thyrotoxic.

The cause of the eye features is controversial. As already stated the minor degrees such as lid retraction or lid lag are due to sympathetic overactivity affecting the levator palpebrae superioris muscle. The more severe degrees of exophthalmos have been thought to be due to increasing mucin and water in the retro-orbital space or due to the myopathy of the extra-ocular muscles allowing the globe to prolapse forward. Accumulations of lymphocytes and deposition of immunoglobulin complexes in the orbital muscles have been postulated as causes of the myopathy and perhaps also of obstruction to the lymphatic drainage of the orbit. Until recently LATS has been implicated in the aetiology of exophthalmos but the support for its involvement is lessening. There is the possibility of there being a separate exophthalmos producing substance (EPS) in the serum of affected patients.

4. In some thyrotoxic patients, especially those with severe

exophthalmos, rather less common features may be seen. These include pretibial myxoedema which is the presence of raised plaques of skin due to deposition of mucin, classically found over the lower third of the legs. These plaques are reddish in colour and have coarse hair associated with them. This condition responds to local steroids—either cream applied under an occlusive dressing or by intradermal injections.

Another feature is thyroid acropathy which resembles finger clubbing and is often associated with deposition of new bone in the phalanges giving an appearance of spindling of the fingers. The characteristic nail change of thyrotoxicosis is onycholysis where there is loss of attachment of the terminal part of the nail to the nail bed.

In some patients a severe chronic myopathy may be present. Characteristically this is a proximal myopathy affecting the gluteal and the deltoid muscles making it difficult for patients to raise their arms or walk upstairs. Much less commonly an acute myopathy which can affect the muscles of the pharynx and larynx may be found.

Methods of diagnosis. In the type of florid case described above the diagnosis essentially is a clinical one and laboratory tests are only confirmatory. The main problem in the diagnosis of thyrotoxicosis is, however, the differential diagnosis of lesser degrees of thyrotoxicosis from patients with an anxiety state who have an incidental small goitre. Usually the experienced clinician can do this readily on clinical examination. Since the treatment of thyrotoxicosis does involve a prolonged period of medical treatment or the possibility of a surgical operation or radio-iodine therapy one should obtain confirmatory laboratory evidence before embarking on therapy.

Providing there is no interfering drug administration, the main one in practice being the administration of oral contraceptives, the diagnosis of thyrotoxicosis may be readily made by selecting any one of the standard tests. For this purpose, modern practice has settled in the main on *in vitro* tests of thyroid function and the usual combination of tests would be the estimation of a serum total T_4 and total T_3. In the majority of patients these will give an unequivocal confirmation of the diagnosis. If there is reason to suspect abnormalities in TBG levels, as for example when the patient is receiving oestrogens, a THUT should also be performed. In a small percentage of patients the biochemical picture of T_3-toxicosis occurs, that is, the syndrome in which the features of thyrotoxicosis are found on examination but where the serum T_4 is normal. This discrepancy can be explained by the finding of increased levels of the other major thyroid hormone T_3.

The diagnosis of thyrotoxicosis in borderline states can be

supported by the presence of an abnormal TRH test, that is, the lack of response of the serum TSH to the stimulus of intravenously administered TRH. Patients with ophthalmic Graves' disease characteristically show no TSH response to TRH. Radio-iodine studies are no longer widely used in the differential diagnosis of thyrotoxicosis from euthyroidism but they are still performed in patients who are potentially for radio-iodine therapy.

Treatment. Once the diagnosis of thyrotoxicosis has been reached a decision must be made about the best means of treatment in a particular patient. As a consequence of our ignorance about the ultimate cause of thyrotoxicosis, the treatment of the condition is symptomatic by controlling excess thyroid hormone production from the thyroid gland. Obviously this is a less than ideal treatment. The choice of treatment possibilities usually falls between one of three methods, anti-thyroid drugs, thyroidectomy and radio-iodine therapy. All have their advantages and disadvantages.

Anti-thyroid drugs. These may be considered in two groups. Firstly, there are drugs which affect the biosynthesis of thyroid hormones in the thyroid gland and secondly, those which block the release of the thyroid hormones from the thyroid or interfere with their peripheral effects.

In the first group the main drugs used are of the thiocarbamide type and the usual one used in Great Britain is carbimazole. This is given initially in doses of 45 to 60 mg/day reducing to maintenance doses of 5 to 15 mg/day when the patient is euthyroid. Other drugs in this group are methimazole, 60 $\rightarrow$ 20 mg/day, propylthiouracil (PTU) 400 $\rightarrow$ 25mg/day, and methylthiouracil 200 $\rightarrow$ 25 mg/day. These drugs all block the iodination of tyrosine.

The other drugs blocking thyroxine biosynthesis affect the uptake of iodine by the thyroid. The one used in clinical practice is potassium perchlorate ($KClO_4$) in doses of 800 $\rightarrow$ 200 mg/day although thiocyanates also have this effect.

With antithyroid drugs a period of about 6 weeks is required to render patients euthyroid. Where antithyroid drugs are used it is generally accepted that they must be continued for at least a year and the problem is that approximately half the patients so treated will show relapse of thyrotoxicosis when the drugs are discontinued. Unfortunately there is no reliable way of predicting which patient will relapse although attempts have been made to correlate a good prognosis with return to normality of T_3 suppressibility of thyroid uptake and the disappearance of thyroid stimulating immunoglobulins. It is likely that antithyroid drugs merely maintain the patient's general condition until a spontaneous remission is allowed to take place rather than have any fundamental effect on the disease itself.

As with all drugs there is an incidence of untoward effects. Skin rashes are relatively common (about 1 per cent of cases). The serious side effects are agranulocytosis with drugs of the thiocarbamide group and especially irreversible aplastic anaemia with potassium perchlorate. These are rare.

Propranolol is the most useful of the drugs blocking the peripheral effects of thyroid hormones. This is often used in the initial stages of treatment but has no long term curative effect. It has a minor effect on the peripheral metabolism of T_4 resulting in a smaller proportion of T_4 being converted to T_3. Iodine, which is discussed below, has also a useful although rather temporary effect. Lithium carbonate which has the interesting effect of blocking thyroid hormone release from the thyroid gland has also been used to a small extent in very thyrotoxic patients.

Since the patients are anxious it is traditional to give sedatives. Recent evidence has shown that drugs like phenobarbitone not only sedate the patient but also increase excretion of the thyroid hormones by enzyme induction in the liver.

Thyroid surgery. Surgery is usually reserved for patients who have a large thyroid gland, especially one causing pressure symptoms, or for those patients who have relapsed following an adequate course of antithyroid drugs. The standard operation is a radical subtotal thyroidectomy and in experienced hands the operation is very successful. Depending how radical the thyroidectomy, there is usually a small risk of relapse of thyrotoxicosis, perhaps of the order of 5 per cent. There is, however, quite a significant incidence of hypothyroidism, in some series as much as 50 per cent, and there are other side effects of the operation, such as damage to the parathyroids or to the recurrent laryngeal nerves, both of which are important complications because of their long term effect. Before thyroidectomy the patient receives a course of carbimazole (or PTU) to render her euthyroid and it is then traditional to give 7 to 10 days treatment with iodine either in the form of potassium iodide (60 mg b.d.) or in the form of Lugol's iodine (5 drops t.i.d.). This is given to render the gland less vascular and friable and, therefore, easier to deal with at the time of operation. It should be noted that where potassium perchlorate has been used pre-operative iodide therapy cannot be used as such doses of iodide would overcome the drug-induced block of iodide uptake and so render the patient thyrotoxic once more.

Radio-iodine therapy. In Britian radio-iodine therapy is still reserved mainly for patients who are over the age of 40 years but in the

United States it is much more widely used in younger patients from the age of 25 years upwards. The usual isotope used has been ^{131}I although small numbers have been treated with ^{125}I with similar results. From the patients' point of view the advantage of radioactive iodine therapy is that it is a simple treatment. The disadvantage is that it is associated with a high incidence of long term hypothyroidism. This has reached, in some series, about 70 per cent by 10 years. One other disadvantage is that it takes three to four months to render a patient euthyroid with a single dose of radioactive iodine and temporary use of antithyroid drugs may be required. The high incidence of hypothyroidism is thought to be due to damage to the reproductive capacity of the thyroid cell. So far there has been no way found of effectively treating thyrotoxicosis by radioactive iodine without causing this type of damage. Pregnancy is of course an absolute contra-indication to treatment with radioactive iodine and most people would accept that young children with thyrotoxicosis should not be treated in this manner because there is an increased incidence of thyroid carcinoma when the growing thyroid is irradiated. On the other hand it is generally accepted that even in the young adult relapse of thyrotoxicosis following thyroidectomy is best treated with radioactive iodine because the theoretical risks of irradiation damage are far outweighed by the practical risks of a second thyroid operation.

Thyroid crisis

In a few patients with severe thyrotoxicosis the symptoms can be suddenly exacerbated and cause a critical illness with hyperpyrexia, severe tachycardia and extreme restlessness. This can occur spontaneously especially in association with severe infections such as pneumonia but it used to be more commonly found after thyroidectomy. This is rare today provided the patient is properly prepared for thyroidectomy but is still occasionally encountered where there has been some management problem. It may also be seen in severely thyrotoxic patients given radio-iodine therapy and for this reason some physicians always treat such patients with a preliminary course of antithyroid drugs.

The treatment of thyrotoxic crisis is physical cooling, administration of a beta blocking drug, the administration of iodide and carbimazole to stop thyroid hormone release and sedation.

Treatment of the ophthalmic features of thyrotoxicosis

Minor changes do not usually require to be treated. If there is concern about the cosmetic appearance this can be improved by counteracting the sympathetic overactivity by use of 5 per cent guanethidine eye drops instilled once or twice daily.

If there is exposure and irritation of eyes methylcellulose eye drops will give some protection. Where exposure is more severe, especially where there is difficulty in shutting the eyes at night, a lateral tarsorraphy (stitching together the outer parts of the eyelids) protects the cornea and also has a good cosmetic result.

The treatment of severe infiltrative changes is the most difficult. Most physicians use high dose steroid therapy but often there is a relapse when the dosage is reduced. Radio-therapy, with shielding of the lens, is used on an experimental basis. Where there is a serious threat to vision some form of surgical decompression by the removal of one of the bony walls of the orbit is the usual treatment.

Thyrotoxicosis caused by a single hyperfunctioning nodule (Plummer's disease)

This usually affects an older age group than that affected by classical Graves' disease. In this condition the patient presents the typical peripheral signs and symptoms of thyroid overactivity but does not have a symmetrically enlarged goitre. Instead she has a single nodule palpable in the thyroid region. Usually there are not the eye signs associated with Graves' disease apart from a minor degree of lid retraction due to sympathetic overactivity. In this group of patients cardiac symptoms may predominate.

In these patients the diagnosis of excess thyroid hormone production is confirmed in the usual way already discussed. Scanning of the neck using either radio-iodine or technetium shows that the only activity is confined to the solitary palpable nodule, the rest of the gland being suppressed. If one repeats the scan after a course of T_3 or T_4 therapy one can show that this nodule is not suppressed confirming that it is functioning autonomously. Opinions vary as to the treatment of choice for this condition but it is generally accepted that antithyroid drugs are not likely to be of long term value and the treatment lies between removing the nodule after a course of preliminary antithyroid drugs or else administering a therapeutic dose of radioactive iodine and destroying the nodule. This latter procedure is safe in this condition because the rest of the gland is protected by being suppressed by the endogenous over-production of T_4 and T_3 and therefore long term hypothyroidism theoretically should not result.

Thyrotoxicosis in the neonate is a well recognised but uncommon condition. It occurs when the mother is or has been thyrotoxic and it spontaneously improves after the first few weeks of post-natal life provided the child is kept alive by appropriate antithyroid drug therapy. In most, but not all, of the cases reported there have been high levels of LATS in the baby's and mother's serum and the improvement in the baby is on the same time scale as disappearance of LATS from its serum. More recently LATS protector (LATSP) has been implicated in the causation of neonatal thyrotoxicosis perhaps in association with LATS. The method of treatment is to administer antithyroid drugs and await spontaneous recovery.

Thyrotoxicosis in childhood. Thyrotoxicosis is uncommon in childhood after the neonatal phase, being much rarer than hypothyroidism in this age group. Once the immediate neonatal period is past thyrotoxicosis is seldom found until around the time of puberty. When it does occur, however, it presents a problem in management and probably the best course is prolonged treatment with antithyroid drugs.

Thyrotoxicosis in pregnancy. Thyrotoxicosis and pregnancy uncommonly co-exist. In part this is because thyrotoxicosis usually causes amenorrhoea or at least anovulatory bleeding. It is, however, a common clinical observation that thyrotoxic patients who are not taking contraceptive precautions often become pregnant when their disease is coming under control. There are two schools of thought as to the management of thyrotoxicosis in pregnancy. One method is to treat such patients throughout their pregnancy and the puerperium with antithyroid drugs. One precaution to be observed is that the dose of antithyroid drugs should be kept as low as possible because otherwise the fetus can develop a goitre. It is also recommended that the mother does not breast feed since the commonly used antithyroid drugs are excreted in the milk. Recent work however has suggested that the amount excreted is small and unlikely to have a significant effect on the fetus. The alternative treatment is thyroidectomy which, if judged to be necessary, should be done in the middle trimester as this is the time at which there is the least chance of any pregnancy complication arising.

Hypothyroidism

Several different processes can give rise to thyroid failure:

1. Primary thyroid failure with atrophy and fibrosis in the gland. This is now thought to represent a sub-group of 2.

2. Autoimmune disease of the thyroid associated with goitre formation (Hashimoto's thyroiditis).

3. Post-irradiation or post-thyroidectomy patients. This is now numerically the largest group.

4. Administration of antithyroid drugs or other drugs which

incidentally interfere with thyroid function. The former are of course the familiar antithyroid drugs of the carbimazole, thiouracil or potassium perchlorate type; examples of the latter include iodides and the antiadrenal drug, aminoglutethimide.

5. Severe iodine deficiency such as is found in endemic goitre areas.

6. In childhood, apart from the above causes which are rather uncommon at this age, thyroid failure can arise due to either failure of development of the thyroid gland (dysgenesis) or one of the enzymatic defects in thyroid hormone formation (dyshormonogenesis).

7. Hypothyroidism secondary to pituitary failure.

Clinical picture. The clinical picture of adult hypothyroidism is clear cut in the fully developed case. The striking features in the history are of cold intolerance, mental and physical lethargy, alteration of texture of the skin and hair and troublesome constipation. Other frequent complaints are of paraesthesia in the hands, due to the compression of the median nerve in the carpal tunnel by mucinous tissue, menstrual upset usually shown by menorrhagia in the female patient and diminished libido in both sexes. In the occasional patient a psychotic state, reversible with thyroxine replacement therapy—'myxoedematous madness'—may be found. The clinical problem is that many of these symptoms are individually non-specific and many middle-aged women complain of one or more of these symptoms without being hypothyroid.

On examination of a hypothyroid patient one is usually struck by the appearance of the patient who has dry scaly skin, rather sparse coarse head hair, infraorbital puffiness, non-pitting oedema round the wrists and the supraclavicular fossa and bradycardia. Infraorbital oedema is often marked and examination of the tendon reflexes in severe cases shows characteristically delayed ankle jerks.

The problem in diagnosis of hypothyroidism is that although the fully developed case is easily recognisable, mild degrees of hypothyroidism are much more subtle in their presentation and especially in the elderly the possibility of hypothyroidism must be regularly borne in mind.

A typical case of so-called spontaneous myxoedema has no thyroid enlargement whereas that due to autoimmune thyroiditis of the Hashimoto type usually is associated with a goitre. A careful history of any previous drug therapy should be taken especially in regard to anti-thyroid drugs and also in regard to interfering drugs especially iodine-containing cough mixtures which are associated with a high incidence of goitrous hypothyroidism. One should of course be alerted to the possibility of hypothyroidism if there is a history of previous destructive therapy such as thyroidectomy or radio-iodine therapy directed at the thyroid gland.

A particularly severely affected hypothyroid patient may present in myxoedema coma. This is usually found where the environmental temperature has been allowed to fall with resultant severe body cooling. It is to be distinguished from the more commonly found condition of hypothermic coma which usually occurs in frail elderly patients often with preceding cerebrovascular disease who are exposed to the same circumstances. Both conditions give a similar appearance with cold skin, low core temperature, puffy face and bradycardia.

Diagnosis. The laboratory diagnosis of hypothyroidism in a severe case is very simple and the standard tests of estimation of serum total T_4 and total T_3 will confirm the diagnosis. The TSH is markedly elevated.

There has been recent interest in the possibility of diagnosing very mild degrees of hypothyroidism by estimation of the serum TSH. Theoretically in the case of primary thyroid failure this should show a very early rise before there is any marked fall in the circulating levels of the thyroid hormones. The demonstration of such cases with a slightly raised circulating TSH with no abnormality in serum thyroid hormone levels has given rise to controversy. On one hand this state has been regarded as representing subclinical hypothyroidism with the implication that thyroid failure will develop. An alternative view is to regard this stage as compensated euthyroidism, that is, that the thyroid gland is maintaining a normal hormone output by means of increased stimulation from the pituitary by means of TSH. No long term data on the fate of such patients is as yet available and until such time one cannot really decide which of the above views is correct nor can one decide whether such cases should be treated with permanent thyroxine therapy or whether they should be merely observed until clinical and biochemical hypothyroidism has supervened, if indeed this occurs.

In cases of hypothyroidism secondary to pituitary failure there is typically no increased level of TSH in the serum. In these patients hypothyroidism is merely a manifestation of one aspect of pituitary failure and the clinical features are those of hypopituitarism rather than of hypothyroidism. Estimation of pituitary hormones in a case suspected from the history or from the examination of having pituitary insufficiency will clarify the issue. This is dealt with in detail in the section of pituitary disease.

In the diagnosis of hypothyroidism one must be aware of the fallacies in thyroid function tests in patients with severe non-endocrine disease—the 'sick euthyroid' syndrome. In these patients low levels of total T_4 and extremely low levels of total T_3 are found but there is no compensatory rise in TSH. The explanations for these changes are alterations in the binding of the thyroid hormones to the serum proteins and the impaired peripheral conversion of T_4 to T_3. Thyroxine therapy does not benefit these patients.

Treatment of hypothyroidism. The treatment of hypothyroidism is to replace the deficient thyroid hormone. The preparation of choice is sodium thyroxine; there is now no reason ever to use dry thyroid as this is of variable potency. The dose of sodium thyroxine varies from patient to patient; usually it is of the order of 0·10 mg to 0·20 mg/day. The initial dose is usually 0·05 mg with increments of 0·05 mg every 2 weeks until a maintenance dose is achieved. In the elderly patient or patients with angina treatment should be even more cautious and an initial dose of 0·025 mg is suggested.

The assessment of the adequacy of treatment is primarily clinical and depends on the abolition of the symptoms and signs of hypothyroidism without causing those of thyrotoxicosis. Usually the adequacy of the dose of thyroxine is confirmed by estimation of the serum total T_4, total T_3 and TSH to ensure that normal hormone levels have been achieved. Some workers have suggested using the TRH test for the purpose of assessing the correct dose but this is unnecessary in most cases. In some patients the development or worsening of angina may limit the dose of thyroxine to below that which fully relieves features of hypothyroidism. Often concurrent use of a beta blocking drug will allow a larger dose of thyroxine to be given.

It is not necessary to use T_3 in routine treatment. This is however used by intragastric tube or by intravenous injection, in the treatment of myxoedema coma in combination with rewarming techniques. The dosage is controversial but often is of the order of 20 μg 8 hourly.

Thyroiditis

Thyroiditis is of various types:

1. Acute thyroiditis due to specific bacteria such as staphylococci etc. This is very uncommon.

2. Acute thyroiditis due to viral infections such as mumps has been described but this is also quite rare.

3. Sub-acute thyroiditis of the de Quervain type is a rare occurrence in this country but is commonly reported in North America, Africa and in Europe. The characteristic history is of a patient who complains of the sudden onset of pain in the region of the thyroid, who develops a unilateral swelling of the thyroid gland which

may then proceed to involve the other side. Systemic symptoms such as fever and general malaise are also present. These symptoms gradually settle down over a period of some weeks and usually the thyroid recovers completely clinically and biochemically. The thyroid hormone levels are often transiently raised and the radioiodine uptake is suppressed. Biopsy at the time of the acute process reveals the presence of an inflammatory infiltrate associated with giant cells. The treatment is with suppressive steroid therapy over the acute febrile phase of the illness.

4. The most common clinical type of thyroiditis found in the United Kingdom is that known as Hashimoto's thyroiditis. Classically this presents in a middle-aged female patient who is euthyroid or mildly hypothyroid and who has on examination a moderately enlarged thyroid, around two to three times the normal size, which is diffusely enlarged and often with a well marked pyramidal lobe. The consistency of the gland is hard and often the surface is finely nodular. The diagnosis of Hashimoto's thyroiditis can readily be made clinically and can be confirmed by biochemical tests showing hypothyroidism with a raised serum TSH value, by estimation of the thyroid antibodies and in selected cases by thyroid biopsy.

Estimation of thyroid antibodies has not in clinical practice proved as useful as it once was hoped. The main reason is that patients with thyroid disease other than Hashimoto's thyroiditis can have thyroid antibodies in their serum. For instance this is found in thyrotoxicosis, non-toxic goitre and sometimes in thyroid cancer. Secondly, not every patient with Hashimoto's thyroiditis has strikingly positive thyroid antibodies. Thirdly, the fact that someone has Hashimoto's thyroiditis does not necessarily exclude them from having any other thyroid disease and there is a clinical impression that carcinoma of the thyroid is more common in patients with Hashimoto's disease. The main value in estimating thyroid antibodies is to confirm an already established clinical diagnosis.

The usual thyroid antibodies estimated are antibodies against thyroglobulin which is estimated by either a precipitin test, which is a test of low sensitivity, or a tanned red cell agglutination test, which is a test of much higher sensitivity. The problem with the latter test is that it is often positive when the clinical condition is other than Hashimoto's thyroiditis. The same drawback applies to the other main type of thyroid antibody test which is for antibodies directed against components of the thyroid epithelial cells. The usual test of this type is a complement fixation test for antibodies against the thyroid microsomes and this is commonly positive in thyroid conditions other than Hashimoto's thyroiditis, in particular, cases of thyrotoxicosis.

In practice the main differential diagnosis of Hashimoto's disease is that of thyroid cancer. Sometimes, because of the hard consistency of the gland in both conditions, thyroiditis, which is unduly unilateral, may give rise to suspicion of malignancy and in this instance the correct management is as for thyroid cancer. Where there is a reasonable clinical and laboratory diagnosis of Hashimoto's thyroiditis the usual management is to put the patient on to suppressive thyroxine therapy and observe her clinically. If the gland shrinks satisfactorily on this therapy one may take it that the diagnosis of Hashimoto's thyroiditis is confirmed but if the gland does not shrink then the suspicion of thyroid cancer must increase and appropriate action be taken.

Riedel's thyroiditis. This is a very much less common type of thyroiditis than Hashimoto's thyroiditis. In this condition there is an invasive fibrous process affecting the thyroid gland and extending into the surrounding tissues which causes severe pressure symptoms. The disease is often unilateral initially but frequently spreads to the other lobe. At operation it is usually impossible to perform a thyroidectomy as the fibrous tissue has infiltrated almost like a malignant process although on histological examination only mature collagen is seen. The usual treatment is attempted surgical decompression insofar as it can be performed and on occasion dramatic cure has been found with steroid therapy.

Hypothyroidism as a side-effect of drugs. Apart from deliberate therapeutic use of the antithyroid agents used in the treatment of thyrotoxicosis, hypothyroidism arising as a side-effect of non-antithyroid drug administration is uncommon. By far the commonest example of this condition is that due to iodide which occurs in a significant number of patients who take large doses of iodine-containing cough medicines. In these patients there is a combination of marked thyroid enlargement usually associated with mild to moderate hypothyroidism. Both the goitre and the hypothyroidism are reversible on withdrawal of the iodine-containing mixture and long term treatment for hypothyroidism is not required. There is a suspicion that this condition does not arise unless the patient has some underlying thyroid abnormality which predisposes to it.

Although many other drugs have an antithyroid effect, for example, the oral hypoglycaemic agents, para-aminosalicyclic acid (PAS), oral anticoagulants and phenylbutazone, in practice usually the action on the thyroid is a mild interference with tyrosine iodination which can only be detected on deliberate testing. It is uncommon for drugs other than iodine to give rise to clinical hypothyroidism. One drug which does do this, however, is the anti-adrenal agent aminoglutethimide.

Hypothyroidism in childhood. This arises from two main aetiological causes, thyroid dysgenesis and dyshormonogenesis.

In the first of these, development of the thyroid gland itself is deficient: there may be no demonstrable thyroid tissue at all on examination of the patient's neck either at operation, post mortem or on detailed scanning of the neck but in our experience in the majority there is some small remnant of thyroid tissue found usually in a site along the line of descent of the thyroglossal duct. This can be readily detected on thyroid scanning and on occasion a nodule may be of a sufficient size to be clinically palpable. When the child is hypothyroid or cretinous the finding of such a subclinical remnant of thyroid tissue is not of great therapeutic relevance. When, however, a euthyroid child presents with a mid-line nodule, scanning of the gland is helpful in the differential diagnosis by demonstrating whether or not thyroid tissue is present in the normal site and whether the mid-line suprahyoid nodule is accumulating iodine.

In dyshormonogenesis the clinical picture is very similar no matter which of the various stages of thyroid hormone synthesis are involved (Fig. 3.1). In all stages with the exception of the coupling process there is an enzymatic step and biochemical deficiencies corresponding to these steps have been shown. The clinical picture is, however, similar in that such patients present as cases of familial goitrous hypothyroidism and with one exception the specific type of defect can not be inferred from clinical examination. The one exception is the patient who presents with goitrous hypothyroidism associated with deaf mutism (Pendred's syndrome). This particular defect is associated with a defective intrathyroidal peroxidase enzyme system.

In childhood, hypothyroidism presents in two main clinical categories, cretinism and juvenile myxoedema. A cretin is usually defined as a child with thyroidal failure present at birth or developing within the first two years of postnatal life, that is, during the time when brain development is proceeding. In the absence of treatment one is left with a child who is both physically and mentally retarded and in whom the administration of adequate thyroxine therapy at that point does not correct the defective mental development. It is, therefore, obviously urgent to make the diagnosis as early as possible in postnatal life. The characteristic clinical presentation of the cretin is a child who is slow to thrive, feeds poorly, has a dry scaly skin, the typical bradycardia of hypothyroidism and a characteristic hoarse cry. In the type of cretinism seen in Britain (sporadic cretinism) there is no goitre since the condition is due to dysgenesis of the thyroid. Indeed the neck often feels very empty. In areas where there is a high incidence of endemic goitre one also finds endemic cretinism which is associated with a goitre. Goitrous cretinism is only found in Britain where there is a dyshormonogenetic defect or where the fetus has been exposed to a thyroid-blocking drug—the maternal ingestion of iodides during pregnancy being particularly noteworthy.

In endemic goitre areas one also sees described a condition referred to as neurological cretinism. These are children who show neurological features such as spastic diplegia, mental deficiency and deafness but who are euthyroid instead of being hypothyroid as anticipated. It is not clear whether this condition of neurological cretinism is due to iodine deficiency or temporary thyroid deficiency in intrauterine life or whether these children are merely the spastic children who happen to be born in an endemic goitre area.

The diagnosis of cretinism is readily confirmed by standard biochemical tests which give results similar to the adult range after the first week of postnatal life. If tests of thyroid function are required before this time they are best performed on cord blood as following childbirth the normal neonate passes through a phase of biochemical thyrotoxicosis which interferes with interpretation of the tests. A useful test of thyroid function in childhood is estimation of the bone age. This is characteristically severely delayed in hypothyroidism and in addition the appearance of epiphyseal dysgenesis—a fragmentation of the epiphyses—may be seen. It may be possible by this means to estimate the time of onset of the hypothyroidism.

A different approach to the diagnosis of cretinism has been the routine screening of dried blood spots taken by heel stab in neonates at the same time as samples for phenylketonuria. The tests used have been either the estimation of the T_4 or T_4 and TSH. The incidence of hypothyroidism found in such surveys is around 1 in 6000 neonates. Since hypothyroidism fulfills most of the ideal features of a screening programme, that it is a serious condition of significant incidence which can be detected by fairly simple and inexpensive tests and which is capable of being treated by a cheap and readily available treatment, it is likely to become a routine test in neonatal paediatric practice.

On the other hand the child with juvenile myxoedema presents quite a different clinical problem. These children usually develop hypothyroidism after the second postnatal year. This implies that they will have some functioning thyroid tissue although this is often present in an ectopic site. At this stage in development the main effect of thyroid hormone deficiency is on somatic growth since brain development is finished and it must be borne in mind that hypothyroidism is one of the clinically important and easily reversible causes of dwarfism. These children characteristically do not look particularly hypothyroid and it is only by bearing the condition in mind and instituting appropriate tests in all dwarfs that the diagnosis will be made.

The treatment of hypothyroidism in childhood is by administering appropriate doses of thyroxine. The child tolerates relatively larger doses of thyroxine per kilo of body weight than does the adult. Regular examination and recording of the height measurements and bone development is required to make sure that the skeletal age does not advance beyond the chronological age or otherwise ultimate stunting of stature will develop.

Non-toxic goitre

The term non-toxic goitre implies the presence in a euthyroid patient of significant thyroid enlargement. The term as usually used is taken to exclude patients with known conditions such as thyroiditis of various types and thyroid cancer. Traditionally the condition of non-toxic goitre is divided into endemic and sporadic goitre depending on the incidence of thyroid enlargement in the population. Conventionally, when more than 10 per cent of the population have a goitre it is referred to as endemic and less than this as sporadic. The division between these two conditions may be, however, artificial.

There have been many goitre surveys in different parts of the world over the last century but the aetiology of goitre even in an endemic area remains confused. Historically, endemic goitre has been and still is found in certain mainly mountainous parts of the world, such as in the Andes, in the Himalayas and in Switzerland. In modern times there have also been studies in the Congo, in South America and New Guinea. As a general rule in most areas in the world in which endemic goitre is found there is an associated high incidence of iodine deficiency but this is not invariable. The administration of iodine, often by intramuscular injection, results in the diminution of the goitre rate and diminution of the goitre size but most surveys have not shown complete abolition of goitre after such iodine administration. Over the years other factors have been proposed to explain the cause of endemic goitre—for instance, water pollution, ingestion of plant goitrogens from turnips, cabbages, kale, secondary ingestion of plant goitrogens which have been excreted in cow's milk and the possible goitrogenic effect of other substances such as calcium have all been suggested. It is true to say that we still do not know what causes goitre. No matter which theory one subscribes to, one has to take account of the fact that non-toxic goitre is approximately 8 times more common in females than in males and this would imply that the influence of sex hormones is important.

The clinical problem of patients with non-toxic goitre as they present in Great Britain is first of all to confirm that the goitre is not associated with thyrotoxicosis, thyroiditis or thyroid cancer. This is done initially on clinical examination. In general in young people with a short history of goitre one would anticipate that the thyroid gland should be soft and not nodular although a goitre which has been present for a long time will become more nodular and firm in consistency. One also wishes to assess the degree of any tracheal displacement and to look for any features of possible thyrotoxicosis or hypothyroidism. Biochemical tests are used to confirm that the patient is euthyroid and scanning of the gland is used to delineate any abnormal areas such as an apparently solitary nodule or an unduly firm area. Having decided that this is indeed a non-toxic goitre the management usually lies between no active therapy, attempting to suppress the gland or thyroid surgery. The general experience with attempted suppression of non-toxic goitres with either thyroxine or T_3 or with giving iodine to abolish any possible element of iodine deficiency has been very disappointing.

Surgery is indicated where there are marked pressure features, where the patient or the surgeon has doubts about the possible malignancy of the thyroid and would wish the gland removed, or where the goitre is causing cosmetic embarassment. In the absence of these features usually no active therapy is given and the patient is merely kept under observation.

Thyroid cancer

Cancer of the thyroid gland is relatively uncommon and accounts for only approximately 400 deaths per annum in the United Kingdom. It falls into four well defined groups.

1. Papillary carcinoma
2. Follicular carcinoma
3. Anaplastic carcinoma
4. Medullary carcinoma

Papillary carcinoma is the main malignant thyroid tumour of childhood and of young adults. This characteristically presents as a solitary thyroid nodule often with tumour in the lateral lymph nodes of the neck at the time of presentation. Occasionally the primary thyroid tumour may be so small as to be impalpable and the patient presents because of the lymph node metastases. This feature has given rise to the concept of the so-called lateral aberrant thyroid which is in fact well differentiated papillary tumour in regional lymph nodes. In recent years there has been increasing evidence that radiation exposure to the neck and upper thorax in childhood is associated with a significant incidence of subsequent thyroid cancer of papillary type. Such radiation was at one time used, especially in America for the treatment of an apparently enlarged thymus, but even superficial radiotherapy used in the treatment of dermatological conditions such as naevi and acne vulgaris is associated with an increased incidence of this type of thyroid tumour.

The correct management of papillary carcinoma is surgical removal of any obvious thyroid tumour, performance of at least a total lobectomy on the affected side but preferably including a subtotal removal of the opposite lobe, in view of the fact that the tumour is often multicentric, and resection of any affected regional lymph nodes. The patient after operation requires life-long suppressive thyroxine therapy in doses adequate to suppress TSH production since there is evidence that these tumours are TSH dependent. The prognosis is very good.

Follicular carcinoma is another type of well differentiated thyroid tumour but this is more common in older patients. Again it presents as a solitary thyroid nodule but characteristically it metastasises to bone and indeed these osseous metastases may be found to be capable of accumulating iodine. This is the one thyroid tumour that is amenable to management with large therapeutic doses of radioactive iodine.

Anaplastic carcinoma is the characteristic thyroid tumour of the elderly. At the time of presentation the patient usually gives a history of having had a goitre for many years previously but there often has been sudden enlargement of the gland. Usually by the time of presentation there are marked features of respiratory obstruction and stridor is common. Often an emergency procedure is needed to relieve the obstruction to respiration and to establish a tissue diagnosis. There is a good but temporary response to external radiotherapy and the long term prognosis is very poor in this undifferentiated tumour.

Medullary carcinoma of thyroid arises from the so-called 'C' cells or light cells of the thyroid gland: that is, those cells which produce the calcium-lowering hormone, calcitonin. It was initially confused pathologically with anaplastic carcinoma but on the whole it occurs in a younger age group and is histologically associated with increased amounts of amyloid tissue in the tumour. A variety of somatic abnormalities have been described in some of these patients, such as marfanoid build, neuromas of the tongue and lips, and there may be associated phaeochromocytomas which are often bilateral and which may occur on a familial basis. The diagnosis may be made pre-operatively by finding increased levels of calcitonin in the blood. Since calcitonin is physiologically released in response to a rising serum calcium level this response may be used as a test in suspected patients by giving an intravenous infusion of calcium and measuring the excessive calcitonin response to this. The increase in calcitonin found after oral whisky has also been used as a diagnostic test. Treatment is surgical removal of the tumour.

FURTHER READING

Burrow G N 1975 Current Concepts of thyroid disease. Medical Clinics of North America 59: 5

Evered D, Hall R 1979 Hypothyroidism and goitre. Clinics in Endocrinology and Metabolism 8: 1

Hoffenberg R 1975 Aetiology of hyperthyroidism. British Medical Journal iii: 452, 508

Volpe R 1978 Thyrotoxicosis. Clinics in Endocrinology and Metabolism 7: 1

4

The ovary

In the adult the ovaries are paired organs each approximately 3 × 1½ cm situated in the pelvis attached to the posterior layer of the broad ligament of the uterus. In the normal ovulating woman the surface is uneven due to follicular rupture.

On microscopic examination the ovary consists of follicles in various stages of development ranging from primordial follicles to one or more follicles undergoing progressive maturation. In the fully mature Graafian follicle there is a well marked large single cell, the ovum, surrounded by a clear zone, the zona pellucida, and this in turn is surrounded by granulosa cells and follicular fluid. Following follicular rupture with the release of the ovum, the cells of the granulosa layer undergo striking changes to become the corpus luteum, the function of which is to produce progesterone to ensure that the endometrium undergoes changes to facilitate easy implantation of a fertilised ovum. The stromal cells round the follicle also alter in appearance to form the thecal layer.

During this cycle of follicular ripening, the endometrium of the uterus has been undergoing changes consisting of thickening and increasing vascularisation. When a corpus luteum is formed the nature of the epithelium changes to a secretory pattern consistent with good implantation and embedding of the ovum. If fertilisation of the ovum does not take place, later on in the cycle there is progressive degeneration of this secretory epithelium and shedding of the epithelium with associated blood loss in the form of the menstrual flow.

ENDOCRINE CONTROL OF THE MENSTRUAL CYCLE

We now have a much clearer idea of the hormonal changes taking place during the menstrual cycle as a result of sensitive tests for changes in the levels of different hormones involved (Fig. 4.1). In the follicular phase of the cycle, that is during the phase when the primordial follicle ripens but preceding release of the ovum, there is

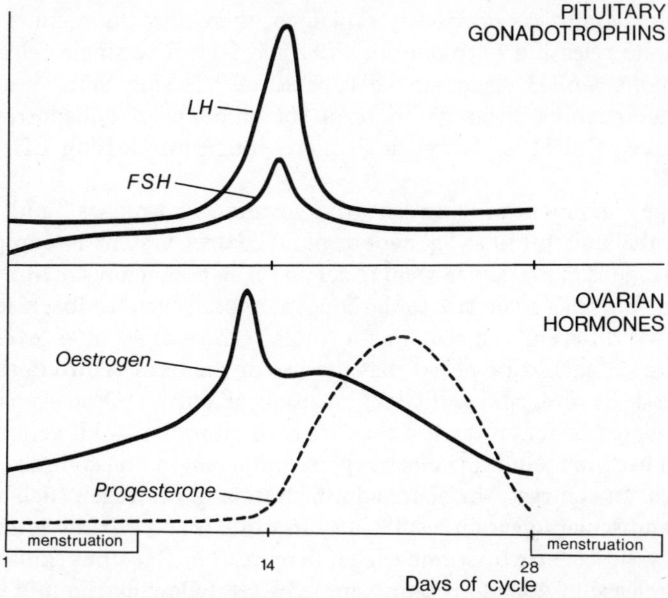

Fig. 4.1 Diagrammatic representation of the endocrine events in the menstrual cycle

an increase in the level of FSH in the plasma. This is what would be anticipated on theoretical grounds. This increasing level of FSH in turn causes an increase in the formation of oestrogen by the ripening follicle. Just prior to the onset of ovulation, that is in the middle of the menstrual cycle or approximately 14 days before the beginning of the next menstrual flow, there is a sudden peak of oestrogen which then shows a very rapid fall. These changes in oestrogen are followed a few hours later by a sudden surge of LH which until this time has been at fairly low levels. At the same time there is a smaller but definite peak of FSH. These gonadotrophin peaks are of short duration and afterwards the levels of LH and FSH fall. In the post ovulatory phase the levels of oestrogen reach lower levels than at the mid-cycle but still remain appreciably higher than in the early proliferative phase. Because of the developing corpus luteum there is a rise in progesterone throughout the latter half of the cycle until the onset of menstruation (in the absence of fertilisation). Should fertilisation take place the levels of oestrogen and progesterone continue to rise throughout pregnancy.

It can be clearly seen therefore that the ovary is under the control of the pituitary by means of release in a cyclical fashion of FSH and LH. In turn the release of gonadotrophins from the pituitary is under the control of the gonadotrophin releasing hormone, GnRH from the hypothalamus. As previously explained, there does not seem to be a separate releasing hormone for FSH and LH. The single releasing hormone GnRH seems to be capable of releasing both pituitary gonadotrophins although in terms of amounts of gonadotrophin released, GnRH is several times more potent in releasing LH than FSH.

The interaction between the ovarian hormones and the hypothalamic/pituitary gonadotrophin control system is complex. Oestrogens in particular seem to act on the hypothalamus in different ways. This has given rise to the concept of oestrogen feedback acting on two different centres—one a 'tonic' centre and one a 'cyclical' centre. It should be noted that the use of the term centre does not necessarily indicate a distinct anatomical entity. Oestrogens are postulated to act on the tonic centre by inhibiting it—this action has been used in including an oestrogen component in oral contraceptive drugs. In contrast, the acute administration of oestrogen such as by intramuscular injection results in a surge of LH and FSH by acting on the cyclical centre by stimulating it to release GnRH—thus explaining the release of gonadotrophins immediately following the mid-cycle peak of oestrogen.

The role of prolactin in the events of the normal menstrual cycle is not yet settled. There is little change in the serum prolactin level throughout the cycle although some workers have claimed to find a small midcycle peak and rather higher levels in the luteal phase of the cycle.

Clinical problems associated with ovarian insufficiency

Primary amenorrhoea

Primary amenorrhoea is the name given to the condition where a female has never menstruated. The age of the menarche is variable in different populations and there is a wide spectrum of normality in individual girls. There is evidence that over the last 50 years or so the age of menarche has diminished to a mean age of around 12 years. It is conventionally accepted that it is not necessarily pathological not to have started to menstruate until after the age of 18 although it is distinctly unusual to go beyond the age of 16 without menstruating or at least showing signs of sexual development.

In girls the earliest features of sexual development are changes in the breast with enlargement of the nipple and areola followed by increasing prominence of the breast tissue. At the same time there is the growth of coarse adult pubic hair over the labia and lower abdomen. These changes progress until the full adult stage of sexual development is reached.

In some girls the development of the breast, pubic hair or onset of menstruation can occur before the conventional earliest age of normal puberty, that is less than 9 years. This condition of precocious puberty has been already discussed in the section dealing with the hypothalamus.

Table 4.1 Causes of primary amenorrhoea

1 *Chromosomal*	–	gonadal dysgenesis (Turner's syndrome)
	–	testicular feminisation (see Ch. 5)
2 *Gynaecological*	–	imperforate hymen and other anatomical abnormalities of the genital tract, ovarian agenesis
3 *Pituitary disease*	–	craniopharyngioma, pituitary adenoma, healed tuberculous meningitis
4 *Delayed puberty*		

Patients presenting with primary amenorrhoea can have a variety of underlying causes. The most important of these is in association with an abnormality of the sex chromosome constitution where there is maldevelopment of the ovary resulting in the presence of merely a 'streak' gonad, that is a small white area of ovarian stroma over the region where the ovaries should normally be. Characteristically this ovarian finding is associated with various somatic abnormalities such as stunting of stature, an increase in the carrying angle, that is the angle which the lower arm makes with the upper arm when the arm is held in the 'anatomical' position, webbing of the neck, a broad 'shield' chest with widely spaced nipples, abnormalities of the fingers and toes including syndactyly and polydactyly, lymphoedema, coarctation of the aorta and the presence of a large number of moles. This spectrum of somatic abnormalities in association with ovarian dysgenesis is known as Turner's syndrome. In the fully developed state this is an easy clinical diagnosis but other patients are seen without gross somatic abnormalities. Certainly any girl with primary amenorrhoea under 5 feet in height should be seriously considered as having gonadal dysgenesis. In such patients it is essential to confirm the diagnosis by appropriate investigation. This can be done by a buccal smear which is a smear made of the epithelial cells obtained by scraping the inside of the mouth. With the appropriate staining techniques, in patients with typical Turner's syndrome there is no Barr body. The Barr body is the densely staining area of condensed chromatin adjacent to the nuclear membrane which is present in normal female (XX) cells. It is thought to represent the normally inactivated X chromosome. Therefore the presumption is that these apparently female patients who have no Barr body have a chromosomal constitution of XO. It is customary also to send blood for karyotyping of the peripheral lymphocytes and using this technique one is able to identify more precisely the chromosomal constitution. By such techniques it can be shown whether there is complete absence of one X chromosome or whether as found in many of these patients, especially those without the somatic manifestations mentioned above, there is a wide variety of different karyotypes. In some patients there are several cell lines, for instance XO and XX—this is referred to as mosaicism. In others a triple X constitution may be found and in yet others there may be more minor abnormalities of the short or long arm of the X chromosome. Culture of other cell lines, for instance fibroblasts obtained by skin biopsy, can be useful when there is a possibility of mosaicism.

Although gonadal dysgenesis is numerically one of the most important causes of primary amenorrhoea there are other causes to be eliminated. One must ensure that there is no simple structural abnormality such as an imperforate hymen. Obviously if this is so therapy is quite simple and consists of surgical incision.

Some females may be seen who have primary amenorrhoea combined with eunuchoid proportions in contrast to the short stature of the patient with chromosomal disorders. In these eunuchoidal patients it can be shown that there is ovarian agenesis, that is complete failure of ovarian development, or the atrophy of the ovaries very early in postnatal life. Oestrogens are the main anabolic hormones in the female and in the absence of normal oestrogen levels epiphyseal closure is delayed—hence the eunuchoidal build.

Patients with pituitary disorders from childhood, such as craniopharyngioma or healed tuberculous meningitis can present with primary amenorrhoea because the damage to the pituitary or hypothalamus has been present before the time of the menarche. In such patients in addition to amenorrhoea and lack of sexual development there may be manifestations of other pituitary disorders such as dwarfism, deficiency of ACTH with secondary cortisol deficiency, and secondary thyroid deficiency from TSH deficiency. The investigation and treatment of these conditions is considered under the appropriate sections.

Numerically however the most common situation is a girl who presents because of failure of onset of menstruation at the 'normal' time but who, on examination, shows normal breast development and normal development of pubic and axillary hair and is of normal stature. In most of these girls the primary amenorrhoea is a manifestation of a delay in the onset of full sexual development without any obvious pathological process being present. These cases demonstrate our lack of knowledge of the normal triggering of gonadotrophin release at menarche and most of such girls on follow-up menstruate and continue to develop sexually quite normally. In patients of this type, once obvious endocrine diseases are excluded a waiting policy should be adopted.

Where there is no immediately obvious cause of primary amenorrhoea, such as gonadal dysgenesis, estimation of the plasma gonadotrophin levels is of value to differentiate between an ovarian and a hypothalamic/pituitary cause. Gonadotrophin levels are increased in the former and decreased in the latter. Primary amenorrhoea due to ovarian failure is not amenable to treatment whereas that due to hypothalamic/pituitary disease may be reversible.

Secondary amenorrhoea

This is the condition where amenorrhoea develops in a woman who has been previously menstruating. There are many physical causes for this, for example:

1. Pregnancy. This must be considered in every female complaining of secondary amenorrhoea.
2. Acquired pituitary disease such as post partum damage, pituitary tumours, especially prolactinomas.
3. Damage to or disease of the ovaries or uterus by inflammatory conditions such as tuberculosis or endometriosis.
4. Rarely virilising conditions of adrenal and ovarian origin.
5. Severe systemic illness such as Crohn's disease, tuberculosis or thyrotoxicosis.

However, in most patients it must be admitted that structural defects of this type are not found. The common clinical problem is to be faced with a patient who complains of secondary amenorrhoea, who is not pregnant and who has no obvious pelvic lesion when assessed by the gynaecologist. Probably the commonest causes for secondary amenorrhoea in this context are either alterations in weight or previous administration of oral contraceptives.

It is very common to find that young women who develop secondary amenorrhoea have been dieting and it is indeed interesting that usually the onset of amenorrhoea coincides with the beginning of the restricted diet and precedes any substantial loss of weight. Since these patients tend to present to the gynaecologist who is primarily interested in excluding pelvic causes of amenorrhoea the diagnosis may be missed unless the question of dieting is specifically enquired into. The mechanism by which dieting causes secondary amenorrhoea without causing marked impairment of physical health is not clear. It is however known that girls with more severe weight loss show endocrine abnormalities in respect to their gonadotrophin response to attempted stimulation with clomiphene (see below). In the more common mild degree of this condition, provided the girl can be persuaded to gain weight, her menstrual cycle will usually return.

An extreme degree of this dietary amenorrhoea is the condition of anorexia nervosa. In this the patient starves herself until she becomes grossly emaciated. Secondary amenorrhoea develops early on in the course of the illness. Previously this condition was confused with other endocrine disorders such as hypopituitarism but both clinically and biochemically there is no evidence of pituitary insufficiency in these girls with the exception of loss of gonadotrophic function and often low thyroid hormone levels. In contrast, the stress hormones, cortisol, GH and prolactin are often elevated. All the evidence points to this disorder being a psychological one. Studies have suggested that the girl's impression of her body build grossly overestimates her weight and certainly such girls continue to starve themselves even when to the most casual observer they are grossly emaciated. Apart from the emaciation clinical examination is usually negative. In particular, the breasts remain reasonably well developed considering the degree of weight loss and axillary and pubic hair is preserved. The psychological state, apart from the aversion to food and the attempts to hide the degree of starvation, is well preserved and most of such patients are not severely depressed and certainly not usually psychotic. In the occasional patient lesions such as tumours in the region of the hypothalamus may become manifest on follow-up, giving an organic explanation for the syndrome, but this is exceptional. Treatment consists of skilled nursing to persuade the patient to eat an adequate diet, and therapy with chlorpromazine to suppress their overactivity. Usually some time at a normal weight is required before resumption of menstruation occurs. Some patients require treatment to induce ovulation to restart the menstrual cycle (see below).

The converse situation, amenorrhoea with obesity, is also quite common. Like the amenorrhoea associated with weight loss the exact mechanism has not been defined but in such patients periods will return if they co-operate in a weight reduction diet.

The other common cause of secondary amenorrhoea in clinical practice is in girls who have been on oral contraceptive drugs. Since the usual combined oestrogen/progesterone preparation acts by causing inhibition of the pituitary and hypothalamus it is not surprising that these drugs can cause suppression of menstruation after their cessation. Usually this is able to be reversed although sometimes stimulation by clomiphene is required. Galactorrhoea is commonly found with 'post pill' amenorrhoea. This galactorrhoea may respond to clomiphene or alternatively bromocriptine, a specific prolactin inhibitor, may be used. Galactorrhoea associated with amenorrhoea may be found in other situations. These are discussed in the section on hypothalamic and pituitary disorders.

Another important cause of secondary amenorrhoea is emotional stress. Where this is severe the diagnosis is obvious but the possibility of a more minor emotional reaction should be considered in other girls especially in those who are out of their normal environment such as students in college or nurses in training. Such patients usually adjust both emotionally and in terms of resumption of menstruation if given time. Patients with more severe problems may need treatment with antidepressants or expert psychiatric help.

Virilising conditions which are a result of adrenal or ovarian androgen production are uncommon with the exception of the polycystic ovarian syndrome (see below). Any excessive hirsutism or clitoral enlargement should be noted on general and gynaecological examination.

In some patients secondary amenorrhoea may occur due to an apparently premature menopause. In these patients one would expect to get other menopausal symptoms such as hot flushes and irritability.

Investigation of secondary amenorrhoea. After having eliminated pregnancy, gynaecological and systemic disease giving rise to secondary amenorrhoea, it is useful to try and localise the level of the defect (Fig. 4.2).

The simplest of these defects to determine is a lesion of the ovary such as premature ovarian failure (level 1). This would be associated with low levels of oestrogen and a high level of gonadotrophins because of the negative feedback effect.

A defect in the pituitary itself (level 2) would be associated with low gonadotrophins and low oestradiol values. Stimulation of gonadotrophin release by GnRH would be ineffective.

In contrast a lesion in the hypothalamus (level 3) with an intact pituitary, would be expected to show low oestradiol and gonadotrophin values which were increased in response to GnRH administration.

In clinical practice it is important to detect patients with secondary amenorrhoea who have ovarian failure but the distinction between

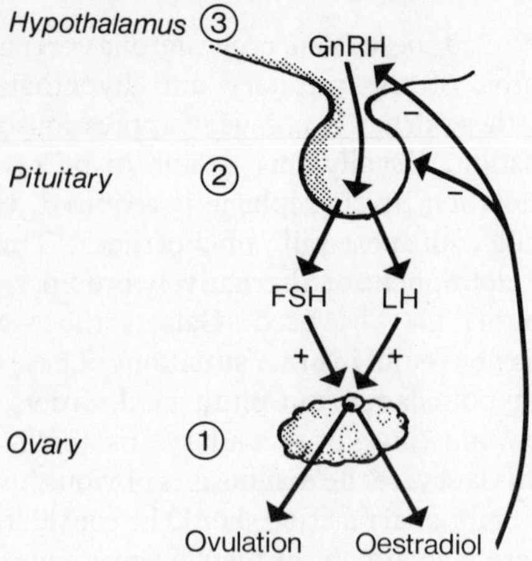

Fig. 4.2 The hypothalamic – pituitary – ovarian axis

pituitary and hypothalamic defects is by no means as clear cut as the above account would suggest.

Treatment of secondary amenorrhoea. Once one has excluded obvious gynaecological or endocrine disease it is worthwhile waiting for some months to see what happens before advocating any treatment. An exception to this policy would be the correcting of an obvious abnormality of weight and treatment of any depressive problems. In many patients spontaneous return of the periods will result. However, on later review of others a decision whether or not to treat the secondary amenorrhoea has to be made. This is usually dependent on the patient's desire or otherwise for pregnancy. If the patient does not wish to become pregnant there is no particular reason to treat secondary amenorrhoea except in those patients who are excessively anxious about not having periods. In such patients it is reasonable to try to induce ovulation with clomiphene but the patient must be warned that she is at risk of becoming pregnant following this treatment unless appropriate contraceptive precautions are taken if these are required.

In patients who are shown to have secondary amenorrhoea due to a premature menopause serious consideration should be given to initiating oestrogen replacement therapy both to prevent atrophy of the genitalia and also to prevent the early onset of degenerative cardiovascular disease and osteoporosis.

Polycystic ovarian syndrome (Stein-Leventhal syndrome)

This is a clinical syndrome of obesity, hirsutism and secondary amenorrhoea associated with enlarged polycystic ovaries. While this is a clinical entity there is doubt whether it is due to a single disease process. There is evidence that a pathological process similar to that found in the polycystic ovarian syndrome, namely ovarian capsular thickening and failure of follicular rupture, can be found where androgens are present in excess no matter what the primary cause of this state. This, for instance, could occur with primary adrenal pathology causing high androgen levels as well as the administration of androgens exogenously. In the spontaneously occurring syndrome it is considered that the ovaries themselves are responsible for synthesising excess androgens in the cystic follicles and that these androgenic steroids are released into the ovarian vein and so into the systemic circulation. There is also the suggestion that adipose tissue is capable of transforming oestrogen to androgens so that by being obese the patient is contributing to her hirsutism.

The clinical diagnosis of Stein-Leventhal syndrome is usually made in the context of finding an overweight, moderately hirsute female who on pelvic examination is found to have bilaterally enlarged ovaries. Usually the periods are either absent or very infrequent. The clinical diagnosis is confirmed by demonstrating the nature of the ovaries either on gynaecography, that is the installation of air into the pelvis with radiological demonstration of the enlarged ovaries, or alternatively, and perhaps more usefully, laparoscopy by which the ovaries can be directly viewed via the laparoscope and a biopsy can be taken to establish the histological nature of the problem. Endocrine investigations will reveal the absence of ovulation. Characteristically the gonadotrophins show an elevated LH with a normal FSH.

Treatment. Until recently this disease was treated by the operation of wedge resection, which is the removal of a wedge of each ovary and the stitching of the ovary together again. This operation was successful in temporarily restoring menstruation and ovulation in a proportion of the patients. Since biopsy of the ovaries at laparoscopy is a basically similar procedure this too can result in the restoration of ovulation. Patients with the Stein-Leventhal syndrome can also be readily induced to ovulate by ovarian stimulation by means of clomiphene or gonadotrophin therapy (see below). Obesity should be treated by appropriate dietary means.

Investigation and treatment of female infertility

The investigations required in the management of infertility in the female depend on what is elicited in the history and on examination of the patient. In some patients it may become obvious from the history that the problem is related to infrequent coitus or to ignorance of coital technique. This should be dealt with by appropriate advice. In a few patients it may become clear on examination that they are suffering from some general endocrine disorder such as hypothyroidism, thyrotoxicosis, pituitary disease etc. This should be dealt with in its own right before any question of treating infertility is considered. In yet another group of patients structural abnormalities such as severe degrees of retroversion of the uterus or blockage of the fallopian tubes due to pelvic adhesions will have been discovered on gynaecological assessment. These abnormalities often result from endometriosis, which is a condition in which there is ectopic endometrial tissue throughout the pelvis with resulting bleeding and fibrosis. This disease may be sometimes amenable to surgical treatment and it does show some response to large doses of progestational drugs and to the antigonadotrophin agent, danazol.

It goes without saying that before taking the investigation of the female very far, especially to the stage of being involved in detailed surgical techniques, one has to be assured that the husband is potentially fertile. This is dealt with in the chapter on the testis.

In women who are amenorrheic there is a prima facie case that the defect in fertility lies in the female and investigations, as outlined above, are indicated. In most patients, however, menstruation is reasonably normal and no obvious cause is found on initial assessment by the gynaecologist and physician and the husband is found to be fertile. The usual investigations in this situation are as outlined below:

1. The patient must be checked gynaecologically to make sure there is no question of tubal blockage. This can be done either by a tubal insufflation test, by passing dye into the cervix at laparoscopy and observing the dye emerging into the pelvis or by hysterosalpingography.

2. It must be established whether or not the woman is ovulating. A variety of techniques are available which are of help in this. These range from very simple techniques such as recording of the basal temperature to complex endocrine investigations.

(a) In the normal cycle the temperature is higher from the onset of ovulation through the second half of the cycle than it is in the first half of the cycle. This is due to the pyrogenic effect of progesterone. If this temperature rise is regularly found the inference is that the female is ovulating regularly but it should be emphasised that this is not conclusive evidence of ovulation.

(b) Tracking studies in which one measures the plasma or urinary oestrogens and progesterone during the menstrual cycle are of great value. In a normally ovulating female there is a rise of oestrogen throughout the first half, i.e. the follicular phase of the cycle, and, following ovulation at mid-cycle, there is a rising level of progesterone in the blood. Such measurements can be performed by measuring the urinary oestrogen and pregnanediol (the main excretory product of progesterone) but with increasing availability of radioimmunoassay techniques it is becoming customary to use estimation of plasma oestrogen and progesterone.

(c) Examination of the endometrium during the second half of the menstrual cycle is of great help in confirming whether or not ovulation is taking place. Where ovulation has occurred the endometrium in the second half of the cycle changes to the secretory type of endometrium and this is reasonably good evidence of ovulation.

(d) Endometrial biopsy at this phase of the cycle may be usefully combined with laparoscopy which enables direct inspection of the ovaries to see whether these have a smooth and inactive surface or whether there is evidence of ovulation as judged by the presence of a corpus luteum which is typically seen as a small haemorrhagic area in the ovary. Even if the patient is not ovulating a laparoscopy does enable the gynaecologist both to test the tubal patency and to perform an ovarian biopsy.

(e) Ovarian biopsy is important in those amenorrheic patients being considered for treatment because it provides information with regard to whether or not there are adequate numbers of primordial follicles in the ovary.

(f) Older tests such as changes in the vaginal epithelium to assess the degree of cornification of the cells are indirect and are no longer used in current practice. One older test, however, which is still useful is a postcoital test, that is, where arrangements are made for a vaginal examination and removal of a specimen of cervical mucus a few hours after intercourse. This allows an assessment of whether adequate numbers of sperm have been deposited in the region of the uterine cervix and it also allows an assessment of the quality of the cervical mucus.

3. In women who have amenorrhoea or oligomenorrhoea an attempt should be made to define which part of the hypothalamic—pituitary—ovarian axis is defective. This has been already dealt with under secondary amenorrhoea.

4. Estimation of the serum prolactin is of value in detecting those patients with hyperprolactinaemia. Some but not all will have clinical galactorrhoea. This has been dealt with in detail under pituitary disorders.

Treatment of infertility

Any obvious general medical, endocrine or local gynaecological condition should of course be treated. If there is tubal blockage attempts may be made to correct this surgically but it must be admitted that the results are poor.

Where there is evidence that ovulation is not taking place and the husband is known to be potentially fertile it is worthwhile considering stimulating ovulation. The selection of patients on the basis of oestrogen and gonadotrophin levels has been discussed above.

There are four main ways in which ovulation can be induced.

1. *Clomiphene*. This is a drug which is structurally like an oestrogen and which seems to be able to block the oestrogen receptors, perhaps in the hypothalamus, thereby causing a negative feedback stimulation of the hypothalamus resulting in subsequent release of GnRH with consequent stimulation of the pituitary to release FSH and LH and therefore the induction of ovulation. This drug does not act in patients who have no functioning anterior pituitary tissue. Caution must be exercised in excluding a pituitary tumour because in such cases sudden enlargement of the pituitary has been recorded. If there is already pressure on the optic nerve this may cause sudden blindness or alternatively the pituitary tumour may undergo infarction with acute hypopituitarism.

Except in these unusual circumstances the drug is simple to use. The usual starting dose is 1 tablet (50 mg) daily from the fourth day of the cycle if the patient is menstruating or starting at any arbitrary time if the patient is not. The patient's response to the drug should ideally be monitored by measuring the hormonal response by plasma assays of progesterone. Monitoring can even be performed by such simple techniques as the basal temperature chart. If there is no induction of ovulation the dose may be steadily increased in each cycle by 1 tablet (50 mg) added per day until dosage as high as 200 mg per day for 5 days may be used. If ovulation is not induced after two or three cycles at this level it is likely that the patient is not going to respond to the drug and an alternative method should be considered.

2. *Gonadotrophin therapy*. This type of treatment started in the 1960's when it was shown that induction of ovulation and pregnancy could be achieved by gonadotrophin extracted from human pituitaries obtained at post mortem. This preparation is referred to as human pituitary gonadotrophin (HPG). Since this was obviously a limited source of material, a major advance in treatment was the isolation and purification of a similar preparation from human menopausal urine which contains gonadotrophins in higher levels than in the menstruating female. This preparation is therefore known as human menopausal gonadotrophin (HMG). It is a mixture of FSH and LH and the preparation most widely used, 'pergonal', contains FSH and LH in a ratio of 7:1. The small amount of LH is not to be regarded as a

harmful contaminant because there is evidence that LH is required for satisfactory induction of ovulation. Using HMG it is essential that the patient should be seen clinically at very frequent intervals and regular laboratory monitoring of the effect of the drug is mandatory. If this is not done the hyperstimulation syndrome may be induced. In this condition the ovaries become grossly enlarged and haemorrhagic. This has resulted in the occasional fatality.

A variety of regimes for administering the drug have been described. The drug may be given in small doses daily or in larger doses on two or three occasions in the first half of the cycle. The effect must be carefully monitored by the oestrogen response. When it is judged that a satisfactory oestrogen response has been achieved, ovulation is then induced by an injection of LH in the form of human chorionic gonadotrophin (HCG). In the absence of the injection of HCG, ovulation will not take place and the changes induced by the HMG will gradually die away. HMG therapy is very successful in inducing ovulation and pregnancy in appropriately selected patients. It is more successful than clomiphene but it does carry a higher risk of induction of multiple ovulation with consequent multiple births.

3. A theoretically alternative method of treatment is to use GnRH. It is possible, provided the pituitary is not destroyed, to induce ovulation by means of giving GnRH instead of HMG. Preliminary evidence suggests that this might be safer in that the pituitary does not seem to respond in an excessive manner no matter what dose of GnRH is used and this may become therefore a safer way to avoid multiple pregnancies and in the future it could come to replace some of the present indications for HMG. It should be noted that treatment with GnRH will not replace HMG in the situation where the pituitary is destroyed.

4. Those patients with hyperprolactinaemia may be treated by selective removal of a pituitary tumour or with bromocriptine if no organic pathology can be shown. This treatment is very successful in inducing ovulation and pregnancy in appropriately selected patients.

Oral contraceptives

The oral contraceptives are the most frequently used drugs which have an endocrine effect. They are of three types:

1. Sequential preparations where an oestrogen is taken for 2 weeks of the cycle followed by a progestogen in addition to the oestrogen for a further week. This is then followed by withdrawal bleeding. This type of preparation is therefore an attempt to closely mimic the endocrine events of the normal menstrual cycle.

2. Combination preparations where a combined oestrogen and progesterone preparation is taken for 21 days followed by one week on no therapy to allow withdrawal bleeding. This is the commonest type of preparation.

3. Progestogen-only preparations.

The initial theory of action of the oral contraceptives was that they inhibited gonadotrophin secretion. However, with the lower dose oestrogen preparations and the progestogen-only pills contraception is achieved without necessarily inhibiting ovulation. These drugs are therefore assumed to act at other sites such as altering the qualities of the cervical mucus, interfering with fallopian tube function and implantation of the fertilised ovum.

The important complications of oral contraceptive drugs are venous thrombosis which may be complicated by pulmonary thromboembolism, occasional arterial thrombosis such as in the cerebral or coronary vessels; hypertension, the aetiology of which is not clear; and hyperlipidaemia due to the effect of oestrogen on a susceptible patient. In addition more minor biochemical abnormalities may be noted on specific testing such as deterioration in carbohydrate tolerance and minor changes in liver function tests. These are rarely of clinical significance. In some patients minor clinical complications such as weight gain, mastalgia, headache and change in libido may be improved by changing the particular preparation. In some patients cessation of oral contraception is followed by secondary amenorrhoea and infertility.

The oral contraceptives are the most reliable form of contraception available. Because they are so widely used it is important that side effects should be minimal. Since many of the unwanted effects seem to be related to the oestrogen content, reduction of this has diminished but not abolished the above complications. It is important to keep in perspective the fact that pregnancy carries with it a higher risk of many of the same complications.

Endocrine treatment of the menopause

There is general agreement that the younger woman who has deficient ovarian function, either from natural disease or surgical operation, should be given oestrogen replacement treatment to prevent premature atrophy of the external genitalia, causing dyspareunia, and to delay osteoporosis.

What is more controversial is the treatment of the patient who has a natural menopause around the normal age of 45–50 years. There would seem a good case to be made for treatment of troublesome hot flushes by short term oestrogen therapy. There is a vogue at present for considering the long term treatment of the post menopausal female by oestrogen therapy to attempt to delay the ageing process. Such treatment will only be justifiable on a large scale if it can be shown that it does not carry an undue risk of the various side effects dealt with under oral contraception.

Ovarian tumours

Cysts and tumours of the ovary are common. Most present to the gynaecologist because of abdominal swelling or are noted incidentally at antenatal, postnatal or family planning consultations. Very few ovarian tumours have endocrine effects. When endocrine symptoms are present these can be either oestrogenic (granulosa cell tumour) or androgenic (arrhenoblastoma and hilus cell tumour). The hilus cell tumour is unusual in that it may produce virilising effects in the absence of significant ovarian enlargement.

The diagnosis of these endocrinologically active ovarian tumours is based on the combination of the clinical evidence of abnormal oestrogen or androgen secretion, supported by appropriate biochemical measurements and the presence of a pelvic mass on gynaecological examination. The treatment is surgical removal of the tumour.

FURTHER READING

Loraine J A (ed) 1973 Reproductive endocrinology and world population. Clinics in Endocrinology and Metabolism 2: 3

Lunenfeld B, Insler V 1974 Classification of amenorrhoeic states and their treatment by ovulation induction. Clinical Endocrinology 3: 223

Ross G T, Lipsett M B 1978 Reproductive Endocrinology. Clinics in Endocrinology and Metabolism 7: 3

Sandler M, Billing B (eds) 1969 The pill: biochemical consequences. Journal of Clinical Pathology Supplement 3

5

The testis

APPLIED ANATOMY

The testes develop from the mesonephric duct system in the male fetus and during intrauterine life the primitive testes descend through the retroperitoneal tissues, along the inguinal canal and into the scrotal sac. In some children this process is arrested and the child presents with undescended testes.

In the adult the testes are organs of two separate functions. Firstly they are the site of formation of spermatozoa and secondly they are endocrine organs by virtue of the synthesis of the male sex hormones. Spermatogenesis takes place in tubules where there is a specialised germinal endothelium consisting of two main types of cells. The first of these is devoted to spermatogenesis and the cells range from primitive precursor cells called spermatogonia which pass through various stages of development as spermatocytes and spermatids until mature sperm are released at the centre of the tubule. In addition to the cells devoted to spermatogenesis other cells are identifiable in the germinal epithelium. These are the pear shaped cells of Sertoli which are thought to have a nutrient function during the process of spermatogenesis.

When the mature sperm are formed they are released into the central part of the tubule from which they pass along through the epididymis into the vas deferens then through the prostate gland, so reaching the exterior through the urethra. Along this complicated course various fluids are added, for example from the seminal vesicles and the prostate. These secretions are thought to have a supportive and nutrient function for the sperm.

The other main function of the testes is the synthesis of the male sex hormone, testosterone. This takes place in specialised clumps of cells, Leydig cells, which lie between the germinal epithelium.

CONTROL OF TESTICULAR FUNCTION

Both aspects of testicular function are under the control of the pituitary and hypothalamus by means of release of gonadotrophins FSH and LH (the latter was formerly referred to in the male as interstitial cell stimulating hormone, ICSH), which are in turn controlled by the gonadotrophin releasing hormone GnRH from the hypothalamus. FSH is concerned mainly with the induction of spermatogenesis through the various stages until mature sperm are formed whereas LH is concerned mainly with stimulating the Leydig cells to synthesise testosterone. This difference in the male is reflected in the differences in the feedback control. It is clear that testosterone exerts a negative feedback on LH release whereas testosterone does not appear to inhibit FSH release. The control of FSH is thought to depend on an as yet unidentified factor 'inhibin' which is postulated to be formed during the latter stages of spermatogenesis.

Assessment of normal testicular function in the adult

1. *Clinical.* A great deal can be learned about normal testicular function from clinical examination. The patient should be examined to see whether he shows evidence of male sex hormone production as shown by the degree of muscular development and by the amount of facial and body hair. The normality or otherwise of size of the penis and testes is estimated, a simple useful instrument for measuring testicular size being the Prader orchidometer, and a general assessment is made for evidence of eunuchoidal proportions, that is undue length of the arms and legs compared to the trunk or of gynaecomastia. The patient should be asked about his sexual function with special reference to frequency of erections and ejaculations and normality or otherwise of intercourse.

If the patient is shaving every day, has normal facial and body hair, shows normal masculine muscle development and is having regular sexual intercourse it can be reasonably assumed that there is no major deficiency of androgen.

2. The *laboratory investigation* of testicular function naturally falls into two parts, (a) the assessment of spermatogenesis and (b) the assessment of Leydig cell function.

a. The assessment of spermatogenesis is performed by simply examining a seminal specimen, obtained by masturbation, with respect to volume of the ejaculate, which should lie between 2 and 5 ml, and sperm concentration. A sperm count of below 20 million/ml on repeated testing is generally accepted as being abnormal whereas counts below 10 million must be regarded as indicating severe loss of spermatogenesis. In addition to the sperm count it is conventional to assess sperm motility, a normal sample having at least 70 per cent of motile forms. It is important in assessing motility that the sample should be collected without use of a condom as this results in sperm immobilisation and thus a false impression of potential fertility.

b. Assessment of Leydig cell function is performed by measuring the plasma testosterone. Testosterone, like many other hormones, is mainly carried in the plasma bound to a carrier protein, in this instance called sex hormone binding globulin (SHBG) which is produced in the liver. The level of free testosterone is thought to be the most important biologically. Variations in the amount of sex hormone binding globulin may therefore be associated with varying testosterone effects. Thus high SHBG levels in male subjects have been described in association with clinical androgen deficiency presumably on the basis of low free hormone levels and normal levels of total testosterone in women have been associated with hirsutism because of a lowered SHBG level resulting in a raised free testosterone.

Assuming no abnormality has been found so far it is likely that testicular function, in both its reproductive and endocrine aspects, is normal.

Clinical testicular disease

Undescended testes

One of the common clinical problems of testicular development referred to the endocrinologist is that of undescended testes. The most important step in the examination is to make quite sure that the testis is undescended and not merely retractile. It is important to examine the child standing, as relaxed as far as possible, and in a warm environment. If neither testicle can be felt in the scrotum the policy to be followed will depend on the age of the child. There is general agreement that is is important to have testicular descent by the time normal puberty arrives but if the child is very young, of the order of 5 or 6 years, it is justifiable to wait for some time to see whether spontaneous descent will occur. Obviously where one testis is in the scrotum one can wait with more equanimity on descent of the other. Before the boy reaches the age of about 10 it is customary to give human chorionic gonadotrophin (HCG). The dose is an arbitrary one but often doses of 1500 to 4000 units twice weekly by intramuscular injection are used for a period of 2 to 3 months. HCG has an LH type action on the testes, that is, it stimulates the interstitial cells to produce testosterone. As the production of testosterone by the developing testis seems to be important in controlling descent of the organ this treatment may be successful.

It is, however, always difficult to say whether, in those cases in which the testes have descended following HCG therapy, this has been the result of the therapy or whether one has merely coincidentally given hormonal treatment at the time when spontaneous change was taking place anyway. In those cases in which testicular descent has not followed the administration of HCG the inguinal canals should be explored and the testes brought down into the scrotum by surgical means if that is possible. Sometimes however this may require such a degree of mobilisation as to impair the vascular supply of the testes with consequent atrophy. It is likely that a proportion of the testes which do not descend spontaneously are intrinsically abnormal.

Apart from the question of improving future fertility, another reason for operating on undescended testes is the more theoretical one of increased risk of malignancy in the undescended gonad.

In some patients with apparently undescended testes, surgical exploration will reveal no testicular tissue (testicular agenesis). Since these patients are of male phenotype it is assumed that the testes have been present in early fetal life, in order that atrophy of the Mullerian ducts should result, but have subsequently been destroyed by some unknown disorder.

Delayed puberty

A relatively common referral is a youth with delayed sexual development. The age at which puberty occurs is variable but certainly it is most unusual for sexual development not to have occurred by the age of 18 years. In most boys with delayed puberty the only findings are of the lack of growth of the penis and testes and absent pubic and axillary hair by the normal age of around 13 years; the stature is short because of the lack of the androgen-induced pubertal growth spurt. In a few of these patients evidence of endocrine disease such as hypopituitarism or hypothyroidism can be found or systemic disease such as malabsorption discovered, but in most no abnormality can be detected. These patients require tests of pituitary and gonadal function. Assuming that no gross abnormality is found, one would usually keep the patient under observation in the expectation that spontaneous puberty would occur. If the boy is 16 years old or more efforts to induce puberty with HCG can be attempted or replacement treatment with testosterone given.

Assessment of male infertility

Assessment of possible factors involved in male infertility is along the lines already dealt with on the clinical assessment of testicular function. A general history should be taken with special relevance to the age of onset of puberty and sexual function. The patient should be asked specifically for any history of disease such as mumps in the post-pubertal period, veneral disease or tuberculous disease which could conceivably result in damage to the testes or to the vas and epididymis. Particular attention should be paid to any local abnormality in the genitalia; testicular size and consistency should be assessed and the presence of any varicocoele should be noted.

A general examination should be made to exclude any other obvious endocrine disease such as hypopituitarism or acromegaly. Assessment should be made of body build and muscular development with a view to assessing whether there is normal androgen production or evidence of eunuchoidal development. Gynaecomastia should be looked for and if associated with eunuchoidal proportions and small firm testes, it is likely that the patient has Klinefelter's syndrome. It should be emphasised that not all patients with an XXY karyotype are necessarily eunuchoidal. Many of these patients are normally hirsute, of normal body proportions and many do not have gynaecomastia. Neither are all males with eunuchoidal proportions necessarily abnormal. Where there is any possibility of pituitary tumour such patients should be assessed by examination of the fundi and of the visual fields, and radiological investigation of the pituitary fossa. It is worth asking about the sense of smell since loss of this sensation is associated with deficiency of the hypothalamic gonadotrophin releasing hormone with subsequent hypogonadism (Kallman's syndrome). In this condition there is maldevelopment of certain midline structures notably the olfactory bulbs and the palate. A subgroup of infertile patients show some of the somatic features found in female patients with gonadal dysgenesis. These include short stature, shield chest, webbed neck and cardiovascular abnormalities. The name of male Turner's syndrome has, therefore, been applied to this group. In the majority of these patients, no chromosomal abnormality can be defined by current techniques in contrast to the female patients with similar somatic abnormalities.

The one group of drugs which should be borne in mind as causing testicular damage comprises the cytotoxic agents. In some patients in whom the damage is not too severe, there may be recovery of spermatogenesis. Radiation treatment to the area of the testes will naturally also result in testicular damage.

Investigation of male infertility. Examination of a seminal specimen is done early in the course of investigation. Where this shows severe oligospermia or azoospermia it is usual to proceed with a testicular biopsy to assess the prognosis. In some patients it will be found that there is spermatogenesis proceeding even though the seminal fluid shows azoospermia. This implies in such cases that there is a blockage between the testicles and the penis. It is, therefore, worthwhile exploring the region of the epididymis to see whether any by-pass procedure is possible. It must be admitted however that the results of such operations are fairly poor. In other patients the testicular biopsy will show advanced disorganisation of spermatogenesis and in some the germinal epithelium will be composed of Sertoli cells only. In others the typical changes of Klinefelter's syndrome will be found with hyalinisation of the germinal epithelium and apparent hyperplasia of the Leydig cells.

In all patients it is important to assess whether infertility is due to primary testicular disease or to primary hypothalamic/pituitary disease (Fig. 5.1). In primary testicular disease one would anticipate high levels of gonadotrophin because of lack of the normal feedback and this is what is found in such conditions as Klinefelter's syndrome,

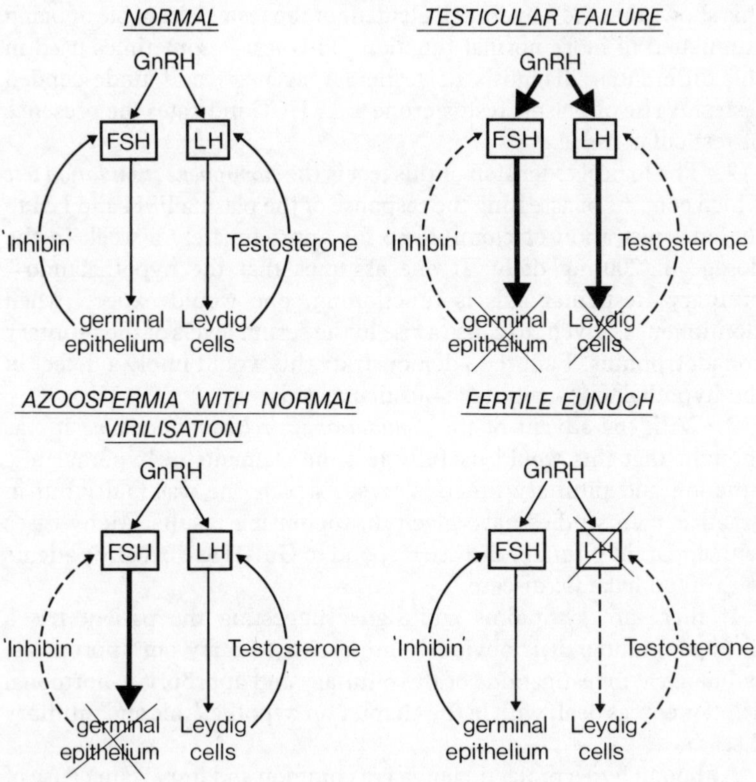

Fig. 5.1 The control of hypothalamic – pituitary – testicular function in health and disease

testicular agenesis, or destructive disease affecting the testes. Where the plasma or urinary FSH and LH are low this would imply that the problem is primarily pituitary or hypothalamic in origin. In some normally virilised males with azoospermia a normal LH level is found because of the normal androgen production but a high FSH level is present because of lack of suppression by 'inhibin'. Some authorities feel that a grossly elevated FSH level indicates such irreversible damage to the germinal epithelium that a testicular biopsy is superfluous as no therapy is likely to be of value. In patients with low levels of gonadotrophins it is important to assess other aspects of pituitary function and it is possible to clarify the testicular problem by peforming dynamic tests of testicular function. These can be considered as follows:

1. *Human chorionic gonadotrophin (HCG) stimulation test.* This depends on the ability of the Leydig cells to respond to the injection of HCG. Where the cells do respond by increased release of testosterone this shows that the Leydig cell element of the testes is capable of being stimulated to more normal function. This test is sometimes used in the differential diagnosis of testicular agenesis and undescended testes. A rise of plasma testosterone after HCG indicates the presence of testicular tissue.

2. The logical extension of this test is the *clomiphene stimulation test* which consists of assessing the response of the plasma FSH and LH to the administration of clomiphene for approximately a week in the dosage of 200 mg daily. If one assumes that the hypothalamic—pituitary—testicular axis is functioning, one would expect, when clomiphene is given, to cause a rise in the serum levels of the pituitary gonadotrophins. Failure to demonstrate this would imply a defect in the hypothalamic—pituitary—testicular axis.

3. With the advent of the *gonadotrophin releasing hormone* it was thought that this would usefully test the elements of hypothalamic function and pituitary function to see which one was faulty but in practice such studies have given disappointing results. Many cases with apparent pituitary disease respond to GnRH as do many patients with hypothalamic disease.

If there are symptoms and signs suggesting the patient has a pituitary tumour it is obviously important to carry out appropriate radiological investigations of the pituitary and appropriate hormonal assessment, as dealt with in the chapter on hypothalamic and pituitary disease.

Although hyperprolactinaemia is a common and important cause of infertility in the female, its role in male infertility is less certain. High prolactin levels in the male are usually associated with large pituitary tumours in contrast to the small and often radiologically inapparent prolactinomas in the female. Partly the reason why small prolactinomas may not be detected in the male is that there is no corresponding male symptom to change in menstrual pattern which is at the mercy of minor changes in endocrine function. The additional fact that the normal prolactin producing cell and also prolactinomas are stimulated by oestrogens especially during pregnancy and when taking the oral contraceptive pill, may encourage the development of such tumours in the female.

If Klinefelter's syndrome is considered likely a buccal smear and karyotyping should be performed. In such patients the classical laboratory abnormalities are the finding of a buccal smear showing the presence of Barr bodies and a karyotype of XXY but in some instances patients who have the clinical picture of Klinefelter's syndrome will be found to have an apparently normal XY karyotyping when performed on the peripheral lymphocytes. It is possible that some of these so-called chromatin-negative Klinefelter's syndrome are cases of mosaicism and that other tissues including the gonad may show abnormal chromosome constitution. In some a more unusual situation may be found where a phenotypic male with the clinical picture of Klinefelter's syndrome may have a 46 XX karyotype, that is the normal female karyotype. With modern techniques it is possible to make a direct identification of the Y chromosome by its fluorescence and difficult cases of this type should be referred to an appropriate laboratory for study.

Since not all cases of Klinefelter's syndrome are clinically hypogonadal, it is important to karyotype all males with azoospermia or severe oligospermia.

There is a subgroup with eunuchoidal proportions—the 'fertile eunuch' who appears to have a selective deficiency of LH with normal levels of FSH. Thus although because of LH deficiency these patients lack androgen (hence the eunuchoidal appearance), they have spermatogenesis although at a lower than normal level. Some of these patients show a response of their sperm count following androgen therapy.

Treatment of male infertility. Those cases which have primary testicular disease are not amenable to any therapy for infertility. The testicular biopsy is of value here in that cases showing tubules lined with Sertoli cells only or cases with severe hyalinisation of the germinal epithelium such as in Klinefelter's syndrome will not respond to treatment. Patients of this type, who in addition to being infertile are hypogonadal, benefit from replacement androgen therapy. This may be given by the oral route but in the long term intramuscular injections of testosterone esters such as 'Sustanon', 500 mg every 2 to 3 months or the implantation of subcutaneous pellets of testosterone in the approximate dosage of 800 mg every 9 to 12 months is preferable.

In the remaining patients any obvious local abnormality such as a varicocoele should be dealt with. Those patients who have obvious endocrine disease, such as a pituitary tumour, will require treatment for the primary endocrine condition in the first instance.

If hyperprolactinaemia is found this will be controlled with bromocriptine which allows restoration of gonadal function, both in terms of synthesising testosterone and in spermatogenesis. Male patients have had both their sexual potency and fertility restored after such treatment.

The male patient with low plasma FSH and LH who shows a response to clomiphene can be given treatment in the long term with this drug in an attempt to induce spermatogenesis. There is evidence, however, that the dose used is critical and doses of greater than 50 mg per day are likely to lead to damage to the germinal epithelium. Furthermore it seems, for an optimal effect, that some LH requires to be given and this is usually administered in the form of injections of HCG once a week in the dose of around 1500 units. Since the process of spermatogenesis takes place over some months this regime must be continued for some time before repeating the sperm count and assessing its response. Experience has shown that very few patients respond but the occasional one does seem to manage to achieve a normal sperm count by this method.

Gonadotrophin therapy in the form of combined FSH and LH ('Pergonal') has also been used in the male but again it is difficult to give a controlled amount of this preparation over a long enough period to ensure adequate spermatogenesis.

Perhaps the greatest hope for the future in this field is the administration of GnRH in therapeutic amounts. This requires to be given by injection on an 8 hourly basis in the dosage of 500 μg 3 times daily. Given in this way there is evidence that GnRH not only stimulates release of FSH and LH from the pituitary but also stimulates synthesis of these hormones within the gland. Following treatment with this preparation there have been several instances of restoration of sexual and reproductive function in the male. One problem about this treatment is that it is very expensive. The development of new longer acting GnRH analogues which will be active by the transnasal route is a possible future therapy.

Impotence

Loss of sexual function in the male is a common cause of referral to the endocrinologist. It is one of the truisms of endocrinology that males with hypogonadism do not usually complain spontaneously of impotence but obviously will admit this symptom on direct questioning. In most men complaining of impotence there are no abnormal physical findings and the symptom commonly presents in the middle-aged male who is driven by his wife to seek medical advice rather against his will. It is frequently found in these patients that the symptom of impotence is a presenting feature of a depressive illness and is not unusually associated with excessive intake of alcohol. It is of interest now, however, that with increasing sexual 'freedom' more and more young men are seeking medical advice because of impotence which is making them feel inadequate to take their place in modern society.

The one important endocrine cause of impotence to be looked for is diabetes mellitus which may cause impotence by means of involvement of the autonomic nervous system. In some males impotence has been the presenting feature of hyperprolactinaemia. Although uncommon it would be important to detect this condition as it is amenable to treatment.

Treatment. The treatment of impotence is very difficult since usually there is no obvious underlying physical disease. The patient should be examined and reassured and any current psychological problems such as endogenous depression should be treated. Hyperprolactinaemia should be treated with bromocriptine. In the normally virilised male use of androgen cannot be recommended in the long term although it is possible that they may give short term psychological benefit to the patient.

Endocrine aspects of testicular tumours

Most testicular tumours present because of enlargement of one testis often associated with some local discomfort. The great majority of testicular tumours arise from the germinal epithelium and of these the most common is the seminoma which is not usually associated with any endocrine effects. The only one of the germinal tumours to show regular endocrine effects is the chorioepithelioma which is commonly associated with gynaecomastia. Like the corresponding tumour in the female the chorioepithelioma is associated with increased levels of human chorionic gonadotrophin (HCG) in the blood and urine. Estimation of HCG can therefore be used both as a diagnostic aid and for assessment of the response to therapy.

Rarely, tumours of the Leydig cells may be found and these can be either androgen- or oestrogen-producing. Increased levels of androgen or oestrogen can be found in the blood and urine. Differentiation from adrenal disease is based on the presence of a testicular mass, adrenal suppression tests and radiology if the diagnosis is in doubt.

FURTHER READING

Butt W R, London D R (eds) 1975 The testes. Clinics in Endocrinology and Metabolism 4: 3

Hendry W F 1979 Male infertility. British Journal of Hospital Medicine 22: 47

6

Disorders of sexual differentiation

INTRODUCTION

Although most people think that they know exactly what is meant by male and female there is in fact no legal definition of sex. The control of sexual development is a very complex process dependent on the full integration of chromosomal constitution, gonadal development, endocrine development, brain development and last but by no means least psychosocial development. These various factors are all inter-related and interact with each other.

CHROMOSOMAL CONSTITUTION

In all normal human individuals there are in each cell, with the exception of the germ cells, 23 pairs of chromosomes. 22 of these pairs are autosomes and the 23rd pair are the sex chromosomes. In the normal female cell there are two X chromosomes giving a 46 XX constitution and in the normal male cell one X chromosome and one Y chromosome giving a 46 XY constitution. The presence of the Y chromosome seems to be a very important determinant of sexual development and except in very rare instances there is no formation of male external genitalia in its absence. Where there is more than one X chromosome associated with a Y chromosome, e.g. 47 XXY, 48 XXXY, 49 XXXXY, the phenotypic development is male. The mature sperm and ovum are different in that they only contain one set of 23 chromosomes. This is as the result of the process of reduction division (meiosis).

The chromosomes cannot be visualised except by special procedures such as the use of drugs like colchicine which arrest the process of cell division at a point where the pairs of chromosomes are in the process of dividing. In appropriate preparations the individual chromosomes are seen to be composed of two strands of chromatin tissue—one of which is destined for each daughter cell; they are joined at one point, the centromere. The chromosomes are classified on the basis of size, position of the centromere, and by the pattern of bands produced by staining with Giemsa stain and other techniques.

In the process of cell division mistakes in transmission of the chromatin strands can result causing either an excess or deficiency of chromatin material in the daughter cell and subsequent generations of cells. Where an autosome is affected major disease is produced, for example mongolism (trisomy 21) and other syndromes often incompatible with life.

Where the sex chromosomes are involved in such a process a more benign phenotypic abnormality is produced. Such syndromes may be associated with additional sex chromatin material such as 47 XXY (Klinefelter's syndrome) which results typically in a hypogonadal male phenotype or 47 XXX syndrome in which a virtually normal female phenotype may be found.

On the other hand there may be a deficiency of chromatin material such as in 45 XO which gives the clinical picture known as Turner's syndrome (see Ch. 4). It would appear that two X chromosomes are required for ovarian development. XO patients virtually always have only streak ovaries with no formation of ovarian follicles. It is thought that the chromosome constitution of 45 YO is incompatible with life as it has never been found in fetal or postnatal material.

In addition to these abnormal chromosome divisions resulting in the addition or deletion of one whole chromosome, a variant may be encountered in which the X chromosome divides transversely instead of longitudinally resulting in the formation of an X chromosome composed of two long arms or alternatively of two short arms. This is referred to as an isochromosome. Minor variants also occur where there are deletions of part of either the short or long arm of the X chromosomes. Sometimes the whole chromosome may be of bizarre shape, for example, a ring chromosome.

In some patients not all cells have the same chromosomal constitution. This state is referred to as mosaicism, for example, 46 XX/45 XO or 46 XY/47 XXY. Mosaicism is thought to result from an abnormality of cell division at an early stage in the division of the fertilised ovum.

It will be appreciated that the nearer the chromosome constitution approaches to the normal state, the less is the phenotypic abnormality produced.

GENITAL DEVELOPMENT

In early fetal life the fetus destined to be male and the fetus destined to be female both possess the Wolffian system of ducts, which form the accessory sexual organs such as the vas deferens, epididymis and seminal vesicles in the male and the Mullerian system of ducts which form the fallopian tubes, the uterus and the upper two-thirds of the vagina in the female. In the course of normal sexual development there is atrophy of the inappropriate duct system thus allowing the correct formation of the internal sexual organs. The factors controlling this differential development are not fully understood but certainly the direction of sexual development seems to depend on the type of gonad that is present. The presence of testicular tissue appears to be responsible for causing atrophy of the Mullerian duct system. The substance concerned does not seem to be testosterone. Its influence is local: in the case of a true hermaphrodite, who may have testicular tissue in one side and ovarian tissue in the other, the Wolffian duct system will develop on the side where the testicular tissue is situated and the Mullerian duct system on the side of the ovary.

ENDOCRINE DEVELOPMENT

The development of the external genitalia is under control of the endocrine system, especially in the male where the production of androgen is essential for the development of the penis and probably also for descent of the testes. In the absence of androgen the external genitilia are of undifferentiated, i.e. female, type.

BRAIN DEVELOPMENT

The gonad is under the control of the anterior pituitary by means of the gonadotrophic hormones, FSH and LH which are controlled by the hypothalamic releasing hormone GnRH. It has also been suggested that the small amount of testosterone present in the male fetus has the effect of altering the brain and particularly hypothalamic function thereafter.

PSYCHOSOCIAL DEVELOPMENT

There is evidence that the psychological sex becomes imprinted very early in social development. It is therefore very important in the case of any sexual ambiguity at birth that the correct decision about the child's sex should be made as early as possible and its upbringing determined accordingly.

Clinical syndromes

Ambiguous sexual development at birth

As a routine, all children when they are born are inspected for congenital abnormalities and this includes inspection of the external genitalia. Thus the appearance at birth is one of the common early starting points in the investigation of abnormalities of sexual development. As already emphasised it is important to make the correct decision about the sex of the child as early as possible to avoid any later complications. With modern techniques one should be able to make the correct decision. The important conditions to be established are (1) the chromosomal sex and (2) the presence or absence of any endocrine abnormality.

1. The chromosomal sex can be readily established by examination of a buccal smear for the presence or absence of sex chromatin (Barr body) on the nuclear membrane. When the Barr body is present it indicates that the chromosomal sex is likely to be 46 XX, i.e. normal female. On occasions two sex chromatin bodies may be seen, i.e. presumptive 47 XXX. Where no sex chromatin is seen the diagnosis is either presumptive 46 XY, normal male, or 45 XO, gonadal dysgenesis.

The results of the buccal smear should be confirmed by karyotyping procedures. These are usually performed on the peripheral lymphocytes in the first instance but fibroblast cultures from skin biopsies can also be used. These techniques enable each chromosome to be identified. Recent advances such as identification of individual chromosomes by the banding pattern and identification of the Y chromosome by fluorescent techniques have simplified the task.

2. The important endocrine abnormality to be excluded is the production of excess androgenic steroids. Examination of the urinary and plasma steroids will permit confirmation of excess androgen production which would strongly suggest the presence of one of the enzymatic defects of cortisol metabolism and in expert hands will delineate the particular type of defect.

Female pseudohermaphrodism

The condition of female pseudohermaphrodism exists where the chromosomal sex is normal female, i.e. 46 XX, the gonads are ovaries but the external genitalia are ambiguous with masculinising features such as clitoral hypertrophy and fusion of the labia. The most important variety of female pseudohermaphrodism is that due to congenital adrenal hyperplasia. These children with ambiguous sexual development as a result of androgen excess of adrenal origin can be readily separated off as they have a chromosomal constitution of 46 XX, i.e. normal female, and have evidence of an excess amount of androgen. As has been emphasised in the chapter on adrenal disease it is important that these defects are diagnosed early not only because one can prevent progressive virilisation of a female child but also because treatment is essential to normal development and even life.

Occasionally anomalous development of the external genitalia of a female fetus may result from the administration to the mother of drugs which have an androgenic effect. Progesterone derivatives which were formerly much used in the treatment of habitual abortion were particularly noteworthy in this respect. These children, therefore, are examples of female pseudohermaphrodism but usually of a clinically mild degree.

Male pseudohermaphrodism

This term indicates the situation where the chromosomal sex is normal male, i.e. 46 XY, the gonads are testes but the external genitalia are ambiguous with features suggestive of female type of development.

Some male children will be found to have a major structural abnormality of their external genitalia such as severe degrees of hypospadias. This defect implies some deficiency of testosterone effect during fetal life. It is often associated with undescended testes and requires plastic surgery to correct the genital abnormality. Sometimes such disorders may be familial. Usually no clinical evidence of systemic endocrine disease is present with the exception of gynaecomastia in some clinical varieties. These chromosomally male children with improperly developed external genitalia may therefore also be classified as male pseudohermaphrodites. In some of these patients biochemical evidence of defective testosterone synthesis from enzyme deficiency in the testes may be found on detailed study.

Recent work has suggested that some tissues such as the genitalia are not responsive to testosterone but require its conversion to dihydroxytestosterone. This would explain cases of male pseudohermaphrodism who apparently lack the androgen effect on the genitalia during fetal life but who virilise normally at puberty under the influence of their endogenous testosterone.

It should be noted that not all children with an enzymatic defect in cortisol synthesis produce excessive androgens. In some where the defect is early on in the pathway there may be defective production of both cortisol and androgens (both in the adrenal and testes) thus resulting in feminisation of the external genitalia of a chromosomally male fetus, that is one variety of male pseudohermaphrodism.

Testicular feminisation. This is a well recognised although uncommon variety of male pseudohermaphrodism where a phenotypic female is found to have amenorrhoea and on investigation is discovered to have a normal male chromosomal constitution of 46 XY. The characteristic physical findings in these patients are that they are tall, have good breast development but characteristically have virtually absent pubic and axillary hair. The external genitalia are female but the vagina is short and blind-ending and there is no uterus. Often bilateral labial swellings are present which are sometimes mistaken for herniae but at operation are found to be testes. In these patients there would seem to be a true end organ unresponsiveness since they do not virilise even when given potent androgen preparations. It is customary to remove the testes once puberty has occurred in view of the possible risks of tumour formation in undescended testes and to rear them as girls. Supplemental oestrogen therapy is required following gonadectomy. There is a subgroup of this disorder with evidence of 'virilisation' such as hirsutism and enlarged clitoris.

Pure gonadal dysgenesis

Some female patients fail to menstruate and are discovered at operation or laparoscopy to have streak gonads reminiscent of gonadal dysgenesis. On karyotyping of these patients it is found that there is no abnormality and a normal 46 XX constitution is present. It is assumed in these patients that there is a limited chromosomal abnormality affecting the gonad only which shows dysgenesis. The analogous situation of testicular agenesis is sometimes seen in the male. Since patients of this group lack the main anabolic hormone appropriate to their sex there usually are eunuchoidal features present, that is, the limbs are unduly long in proportion to the body. High gonadotrophin levels are found in these patients since their defects are examples of end organ failure.

True hermaphrodism

This term implies the presence in the same individual of both ovarian and testicular tissue. A complex mixture of abnormalities of the external and internal genitalia may be found with often a mixed development of both Mullerian and Wolffian duct systems. Often there is testicular tissue on one side and ovarian tissue on the other but sometimes a mixed gonad containing both ovarian and testicular tissue is produced (ovotestis). The chromosomal sex is variable but is most frequently 46 XX.

Abnormal sexual development at puberty or in the adult patient

Major changes in the sex chromatin constitution such as Klinefelter's syndrome or Turner's syndrome (see chapter on testis and ovary respectively) often are not diagnosed until the time of puberty. This is because the external genitalia are not significantly abnormal for the pre-pubertal child. What is abnormal is the lack of development of the normal secondary sex characteristics at puberty.

In addition in some female patients minor defects in adrenal enzyme function may not become manifest until around puberty. Likewise the development of an androgen secreting tumour in a female after the age of puberty will result in the clinical features of androgen excess such as hirsutism and clitoral enlargement. It should be noted that there is no fusion of the labia in these patients as this will only result where the child has been exposed to excessive androgen before completion of development of the external genitalia, that is, up to 12 weeks of fetal life.

Problems encountered in dealing with ambiguous sexual development in the older child or in the adult

Where there has been either a missed diagnosis or an incorrect diagnosis one may be faced with the problem of dealing with an older child or adult with abnormal sexual development. These cases are difficult to handle and one must take the whole clinical picture into account and not make the decision about allocating sex only on the basis of one facet such as the chromosomal constitution. One very important aspect which must be carefully considered is the state of development of the external genitalia. It is usually much more difficult to construct satisfactory external male genitalia than external female genitalia and therefore unless there is overwhelming psychosocial development towards the male side it is better not to try and masculinise the external genitalia by surgery. This can on occasions, however, be performed even in the author's experience in a chromosomally female (46 XX) patient with very severe virilisation from the adrenogenital syndrome in whom the diagnosis was missed until adult life. The psychological sex was strongly male and therefore it was decided to attempt to improve the external genitalia by surgery. It was possible in this patient to correct the apparent hypospadias and construct acceptable male genitalia. Such patients would of course be infertile as 'males' although theoretically would be capable of ovulating.

The alternative procedure, namely to remove the enlarged clitoris and to open the mid-line perineal tissues and construct, if necessary, an artificial vagina, is a simpler procedure and is performed in those cases with marked virilisation of the external genitalia who are to be reared as females. It should be remembered that patients with the adrenogenital syndrome have normal ovaries and are potentially and indeed in practice fertile provided their genitalia can be reconstructed to allow them to have normal intercourse and provided that they are given therapy with hydrocortisone in amounts sufficient to suppress their adrenal androgen over-production. Since they are affected by an inherited disease appropriate genetic advice should be offered. It is obvious that any patients in whom a procedure is performed which alters the sexual status in which he or she has been reared should receive most careful psychological and endocrine follow-up.

Sex 'reversal' in the physically normal individual

There has been some interest and notoriety in 'sex change' operations in physically normal individuals. In these individuals, both male and female, there is no physical or endocrine abnormality, the disorder being entirely that of psychosexual adjustment. In some of these patients it will be found that they have been taking hormones to promote their physical development towards that of their desired sex, for instance taking oestrogen to promote breast development. The decision about the correct treatment for these patients is extremely difficult. They are certainly unhappy individuals and it may be that in some it is justifiable to consider some operative procedure and appropriate sex hormone therapy where the degree of identification with the sex different from their natural sex is so extreme as to prevent any normal life in their natural role. Such procedures should only be taken after the most careful consideration and consultation between the endocrinologist and the psychiatrist and after an appropriate period of observation.

7

Disturbances of carbohydrate metabolism

The pancreas is a derivative of the foregut and this organ serves two functions, exocrine to produce the pancreatic secretion containing bicarbonate and digestive enzymes, and endocrine to produce the hormones insulin and glucagon. These endocrine functions are associated with special foci of cells called the islets of Langerhans. On microscopic examination of islet tissue one can by special stains identify four different types of cell, the alpha cell, which is the source of glucagon, the beta cell which is the source of insulin, the delta cell which is capable of producing somatostatin and the D_1cell (type 4) which is thought to produce pancreatic polypeptide. The clinical syndromes associated with abnormalities of glucagon, gastrin and somatostatin secretion are dealt with in the chapter on gastrointestinal hormones.

CONTROL OF BLOOD SUGAR AND INSULIN SECRETION

The main physiological control of insulin secretion is its response to the circulating blood sugar. It can readily be shown that following a carbohydrate-containing meal there is a rise in insulin secretion which occurs concurrently with the rise in plasma glucose and falls off with a similar time scale. The important physiological action of insulin appears to be to increase the uptake of glucose into the peripheral tissues and also into the liver where it stimulates the formation of glycogen. It also stimulates the formation of protein and lipid and therefore is one of the most important of the anabolic hormones.

In addition to its physiological control by the blood sugar, insulin also is influenced by many different hormones. Important amongst these is growth hormone which has a potent stimulatory effect on the islet cell tissue. In excess, this may eventually lead to exhaustion atrophy of the islet cell tissue. Carbohydrate intolerance is therefore commonly encountered in acromegaly. In addition to growth hormone, the glucocorticoids produced by the adrenal have, as their name would suggest, important effects on carbohydrate metabolism.

They have a tendency to cause diabetes mellitus by means of breakdown of liver glycogen (glycogenolysis) and promoting the formation of glucose from protein (gluconeogenesis). Thus hyperglycaemia is a common finding where glucocorticoids are produced in excess as in spontaneously occurring Cushing's syndrome or during the administration of exogenous glucocorticoids. Thyroid hormones also play a part in the regulation of carbohydrate metabolism by promoting glycogen breakdown, and thus hyperglycaemia and glycosuria which are reversible by controlling the thyroid overactivity may be found in thyrotoxicosis. In addition, other hormones have a more minor role including, paradoxically, glucagon whose main action is to raise the blood sugar. This hormone has been shown under certain circumstances to stimulate insulin secretion. Adrenaline promotes hyperglycaemia by inhibiting insulin release from the islet tissue and also by promoting glycogenolysis.

The level of blood sugar found at any point in time is the result of an equilibrium between glucose absorption from the gut, glucose uptake into the peripheral tissue such as muscle or brain, the formation of glycogen in the liver (glycogenesis), the breakdown of liver glycogen (glycogenolysis), the formation of glucose from pyruvate and lactate (glucogenesis),' the formation of glucose from amino acids (gluconeogenesis) and the interaction with fat metabolism especially with the free fatty acid fraction of the plasma which can be used by many tissues as an alternative source of energy to glucose.

Clinical types of diabetes mellitus

These are conventionally grouped under the following headings:

1. *Potential,* which is the condition where the patient has a congenital predisposition to develop diabetes. Such patients may for instance have a very strong family history of diabetes or be one of two identical twins, the other of whom has already developed diabetes. In females where there is a history of having had large babies (over 4·5 kg) there is a strong tendency to develop diabetes in later life. It is obvious that in this miscellaneous group of conditions there can be no certainty about the development of diabetes until the person has gone on to manifest more obvious diabetic abnormalities.

2. *Latent diabetes.* This term is used to describe individuals who are otherwise normal but who under certain conditions of stress or following the administration of steroids develop abnormalities of carbohydrate tolerance with glycosuria and hyperglycaemia.

3. *Asymptomatic diabetes* is the condition where a patient is found, incidentally, often as the result of an insurance examination or a routine visit to a hospital outpatient department with an incidental illness, to have glycosuria and hyperglycaemia.

4. *Clinical diabetes* is where the patient presents with major symptoms of diabetes mellitus or with overt complications attributable to the disease.

It is recognised in most population surveys in European-derived populations that there is an incidence of known diabetes mellitus in the population of approximately 1 per cent with an additional 1 per cent found on biochemical screening. In certain population groups, however, the incidence of diabetes is very much higher, for instance the Indian population in South Africa and the Pima Indians in North America. Conversely in some ethnic groups the incidence is very much lower. Some of these differences are as a result of major differences in dietary habits and exercise.

Causes of secondary diabetes mellitus

The ultimate cause of diabetes mellitus is unknown in most patients. In a few the reason for the development of diabetes can be inferred from associated disease, e.g. other endocrine syndromes such as acromegaly, Cushing's syndrome and thyrotoxicosis in which there is excess of a hormone which promotes hyperglycaemia, or because of pancreatic disease such as chronic pancreatitis or pancreatic carcinoma. In some patients drugs, particularly glucocorticoids, oral contraceptives and thiazide diuretics can precipitate the condition. Rarely, diabetes may be a manifestation of a generalised metabolic disorder such as haemochromatosis. It is important to recognise these secondary types of diabetes as they may be amenable to cure.

Cause of 'idiopathic' diabetes mellitus

In the majority of cases the clinical disorder of diabetes mellitus would seem to be the result of the accumulation of many exogenous factors such as increasing age, diet, obesity, stress, infections and drugs acting on a person with a hereditary predisposition to the disease. Diabetes, especially juvenile-onset diabetes, has been found to be correlated with certain of the histocompatability antigens especially HL-A B w 8 and HL-A B w 15. This genetic make up may result in a predisposition to autoimmune disease the onset of which may be triggered by viral infection especially of the Coxsackie type.

Screening for diabetes mellitus

Since diabetes mellitus is an important disease with major complications it is imperative that the diagnosis should be made as early as possible and to this end much work has been done to find what is the most effective means of diagnosing early diabetes mellitus. The opportunity should be taken to test a patient's urine when he presents to the hospital outpatient department irrespective of the nature of his complaint and urine testing should form a routine part of all general examinations of patients. To increase the yield of patients attempts have been made to screen large numbers of the general population who are apparently asymptomatic. This has been approached in various ways such as by providing the whole population of a town with instructions for use of a test tape specific for glucose and getting the people to test their own urine and to report when an abnormal result is found. It is important, however, to be aware that the presence of glycosuria itself does not constitute a diagnosis of diabetes mellitus. In many patients found in such screening procedures to have glycosuria, it will be shown that the abnormality is an abnormal renal threshold to glucose whereby the patients develop glycosuria at lower blood sugar levels than are conventionally associated with renal tubular loss of glucose. Other patients will show a lag curve, that is a curve of blood sugar values which reach levels above the conventional renal threshold very rapidly but which fall so that the blood sugar rapidly returns to normal levels. Obviously in such patients glycosuria will result for the duration of the time that the blood sugar is above the renal threshold. This type of blood sugar curve is commonly seen after gastric surgery and therefore glycosuria is a common finding in such patients. There is no good evidence that either a low renal threshold for glucose or a lag curve pattern of blood sugar response to an oral glucose load is associated with a predisposition to diabetes mellitus.

Because of these problems in interpreting urine sugar values, screening procedures have been undertaken which have depended on a single 2 hour post-prandial venous blood sample. In normal individuals by this time the blood glucose should have fallen to levels below 7·0 mmol/l (conversion factor blood or plasma glucose in mmol/l $\times$ 18·02 = blood or plasma glucose in mg/100 ml). Values above this are strongly suggestive of diabetes mellitus.

Laboratory confirmation of diabetes mellitus

The standard procedure to confirm the diagnosis and the one which should be carried out in all patients with glycosuria unless this is gross and associated with obvious clinical diabetes mellitus is the oral glucose tolerance test. This test has been in use for over half a century and the broad criteria of normality have been worked out although there is certain dispute over more minor details. It is generally accepted that the fasting blood sugar should be less than 6·5 mmol/l, that the peak value obtained after 50 g of glucose should be less than 10·0 mmol/l and by 2 hours the blood sugar values should have returned to below 7·0 mmol/l.

There is difficulty in interpreting figures in the literature as earlier methods involved the use of techniques which measured 'reducing substances' including glucose but were not specific for glucose. Now it is usual to use a specific technique for measuring blood glucose. This gives a value about 10 per cent lower than the older methods. A further complication is that in some laboratories the plasma glucose is measured. The plasma glucose is approximately 15 per cent higher than the whole blood glucose. Clearly one must be guided by the local laboratory as to its 'normal' range.

Important practical points are to make sure that the patient has an adequate carbohydrate-containing diet for several days before the test is done and to ensure that the patient is rested for 30 minutes before the test and forbidden to smoke. If these points are not observed, falsely abnormal values may be obtained. Abnormal values may be obtained in patients with renal disease. The situation is complex as both the postprandial blood sugar and the plasma insulin are often elevated, the latter due to failure of the kidney to degrade insulin. Because of this unusual spectrum of results it has been suggested that the failing kidney may retain some, as yet unidentified, insulin antagonist.

It has only recently been appreciated that there are major differences in carbohydrate tolerance with age and with the time of the day the test is performed and so it is important to try and standardise the test as far as possible.

Because of these problems, attempts have been made to develop a standardised test of carbohydrate tolerance based on the clearance of glucose from the blood following the injection of an intravenous dose of glucose. This intravenous glucose tolerance test has not become widely accepted in practice and it is of course not as physiological a test as an oral glucose test. There is evidence that some of the gastrointestinal hormones such as enteroglucagon may have a role in the regulation of insulin secretion.

In some patients who are suspected of having latent diabetes, glucose tolerance tests may be repeated after the administration of small doses of glucocorticoids. This serves to aggravate any tendency to diabetes.

It should be noted that estimation of the plasma insulin does not form a routine test for diabetes mellitus. The plasma insulin responses in diabetes to an orally administered glucose load are variable. In advanced insulin-dependent diabetes mellitus there may be no detectable insulin produced in response to a carbohydrate load whereas in other patients with diabetes mellitus, especially in older obese patients, the insulin response to a glucose load may be larger than normal but it does not occur synchronously with the rise in blood glucose. Instead the insulin response is characteristically delayed and reaches its peak after the peak of blood sugar has passed. It will therefore be appreciated that since clinical diabetes mellitus may be associated with either an absent or an excessive response of insulin this is not a test with a high diagnostic discrimination for the presence of diabetes mellitus. The assay of insulin has additional problems. One of these is that there are discrepancies between the radioimmunoassay and the bioassay of insulin. The other is that insulin is present in a variety of forms which has given rise to a confusing nomenclature. There is a larger molecular weight insulin referred to as proinsulin which is a precursor of the active hormone.

Clinical features of diabetes mellitus

Patients with diabetes mellitus present in two broad categories. Firstly there is the young, usually underweight, insulin dependent patient and secondly there is the middle aged, usually obese, non-insulin dependent diabetic. It will be appreciated that the demarcation between these groups is not strict. The distinction is however clinically useful as it has implications for treatment. Patients falling in an intermediate group are sometimes seen. For instance a group of young diabetic patients has been described with apparently maturity onset type diabetes which is inherited as an autosomal dominant defect (maturity onset diabetes in young people-MODY). Although uncommon it is important in view of its distinct pattern of inheritance.

Typical modes of presentation of diabetes mellitus are:

1. Polyuria, polydipsia and polyphagia; these symptoms often being accompanied by marked weight loss despite the increased appetite especially for carbohydrate-containing foods.

2. Presentation because of infection. This especially occurs in the female where an intractable monilial vulvo-vaginitis is a common presenting problem. There is a certain amount of dispute as to whether diabetics are really more prone to other infections than normal people but it has been suggested that in addition to superficial skin infections they may be more liable to urinary tract infections than non-diabetic patients.

3. A diabetic patient may first present with one of the long-term complications of the disease. Common amongst these are peripheral vascular disease, neuropathy, ophthalmic complications and renal involvement.

Peripheral vascular disease is more common in the diabetic patient than in the non-diabetic. This is due to the hyperlipidaemic state of diabetes mellitus which causes secondary atheroma with resultant diminution of blood flow to the peripheries. Certainly ischaemic ulcers and peripheral gangrene are a common finding in long term diabetes, the disorder often being complicated by an accompanying neuropathy.

The neuropathy of diabetes can occur in many forms. By far the most common is a sensory neuropathy which can readily be demonstrated in many long term diabetic patients. Often this is virtually asymptomatic and is only diagnosed by formal testing which reveals the typical glove-stocking anaesthesia. In patients who are predisposed to develop peripheral vascular disease, the presence of a sensory neuropathy in addition aggravates any tendency to ulcer formation by permitting the patient to walk on a limb which would otherwise be rested, so resulting in a combination of atherosclerotic and neuropathic ulceration. This often starts where the patient has unwisely performed minor self treatment procedures on the feet, such as paring corns or cutting back an ingrowing toenail. From such minor trauma, major ischaemic areas may develop. Occasionally a major sensory neuropathy may be found which may mimic tabes dorsalis especially when associated with pupillary abnormalities of the Argyll-Robertson type—hence the term diabetic pseudotabes.

Another form of neuropathy is a motor neuropathy which is manifest mainly by loss of tendon jerks in the legs on clinical testing. It is also often asymptomatic. Sometimes motor impairment may affect one particular nerve (mononeuropathy), often one of the cranial nerves. Isolated cranial nerve lesions of sudden onset, particularly affecting the 3rd nerve, are well recognised features of diabetes.

Lastly the neuropathy may affect predominantly the autonomic system and this may result in disorders of sweating, impotence, difficulty in micturition, diarrhoea (diabetic diarrhoea) and postural hypotension.

The ultimate cause of the neuropathy of diabetes is not clear. There are grounds for thinking that some early examples may be induced by metabolic changes because the neuropathy appears to be able to be at least partially reversed by attaining adequate diabetic control. In the more severe degrees, however, it would appear likely that the neuropathy is a mixture of metabolic and ischaemic changes consequent on the increasing atheroma of the vasa nervorum.

Apart from the isolated cranial nerve lesions already mentioned, the eye is one of the important areas of diabetic complications. It is recognised that diabetic patients develop cataracts earlier than the non-diabetic. The actual type of cataract is, however, usually indistinguishable from the ordinary 'senile' cataract. Of much greater importance, however, are the retinal changes which can occur. In most longstanding diabetic patients ophthalmological review will reveal changes in the retina. Some of these changes may be of diagnostic significance and sometimes the first diagnosis of diabetes may be made by the ophthalmologist noting the presence of the typical microaneurysms. These appear as little red dots between the retinal vessels but not apparently related to them. Microaneurysms arise from the deep retinal capillaries. In addition to the typical microaneurysms, diabetic patients may show soft or hard exudates and there may also be haemorrhages in the retina. Because these are in the deep layers of the retina they appear as blobs rather than the typical superficial flame shaped haemorrhages found in hypertension. Some of these changes are very similar to those found in a hypertensive fundus. The main differentiating points, apart from the presence of hypertension in the one and not in the other, are that the vascular changes are much more severe in hypertension and that papilloedema is not found in the diabetic patient unless there is some incidental intracranial cause for this.

Most of the retinal changes so far described do not result in any significant visual impairment unless the macula is directly affected, but there is one diabetic lesion which is a major cause of blindness. This is proliferative retinopathy in which there is a growth of new vessels resulting in a tendency to vitreous haemorrhage which then in turn undergoes neovascularisation—retinitis proliferans. Diabetic complications are one of the leading causes of blindness.

Many longstanding diabetics will be found on urine testing to have marked proteinuria and may indeed in advanced cases show the clinical features of the nephrotic syndrome with proteinuria, hypoproteinaemia and marked oedema. At renal biopsy or at necropsy it can be shown that glomerulosclerotic changes are common and in a minority of cases there are specific lesions of the kidney with nodular sclerosis in the glomerular capillaries. This pathological entity is referred to as the Kimmelstiel-Wilson syndrome. In such patients there is renal damage which is progressive and no known treatment is of benefit.

Minor complications of diabetes are related to the skin which is liable to infections with pyogenic bacteria and fungi. Pruritus either localised over the genitalia or occurring more generally over the body is a well recognised feature. Some diabetics who have severe hyperlipidaemia may present to the dermatologist because of multiple xanthomata. Sometimes more specific lesions associated with diabetes are found. Necrobiosis lipoidica diabeticorum consists of indurated yellowish-red plaques found typically over the front of the lower leg, and on biopsy showing foamy lipid-filled cells. Diabetic dermopathy consists of pigmented patches of variable size over the same area.

Patients may also present initially with acute complications of diabetes such as diabetic ketoacidosis. This important condition is considered later.

Treatment of diabetes mellitus

The ideal aim is the complete control of the metabolic defects and the prevention of complications. This is rarely achieved as it is very difficult even with regular urine testing to ensure that the metabolic defect is well controlled all the time and the treatments with oral hypoglycaemic drugs or insulins at present available, although very good, are not ideal. Recently it has been found that a minor component of haemoglobin (HbA_1C) a glycosylated haemoglobin which has had a hexose group added in the peripheral circulation, is increased where diabetic control has been poor. Measurement of this component may therefore be used to give a long term view of the adequacy or otherwise of treatment and may allow better correlation of poor control with the complications outlined above.

The routine treatment of diabetes mellitus consists of two main parts. Firstly, alterations to the diet and secondly, prescription if required of additional therapy to deal with hyperglycaemia.

It is of fundamental importance to ensure that a diabetic patient is put on to a diet appropriate to his body weight and calorie expenditure. In deciding what diet is most suitable the help of a skilled dietician is most useful but is not absolutely essential. A variety of dietary regimes has been described ranging from diets which only restrict carbohydrate to diets which require careful measurement of all the dietary constituents. It is obvious that the less complicated the dietary regime is and the least removed it is from ordinary eating habits the more likely the patient will cooperate in the long term.

The group who are theoretically most simple to treat is the overweight, maturity-onset diabetic. As a general rule these patients have an excessive insulin response to hyperglycaemia so they do not require insulin for routine treatment. They respond well to weight reduction coupled with carbohydrate restriction. Although a regime of this type apparently is simple for the patient to follow, it must be acknowledged that it is very difficult to persuade many patients, especially those who are virtually asymptomatic, to follow a proper weight reduction diet.

In the typical young, thin, insulin dependent diabetic who has a tendency to ketosis, diet is also important. It is essential to make sure that the diet in these patients contains an adequate amount of calories and of carbohydrate. The amount of carbohydrate in the diet is one of the major factors in deciding the insulin requirements. It is important, however, not to attempt to control these patients by excessively reducing their carbohydrate intake as this will aggravate the ketosis by causing mobilisation of fat instead of carbohydrate. The calorie requirement of such a patient depends on his occupation and the degree of weight loss. For instance, for an average sedentary occupation, many patients will remain well on something of the order of 1500–2000 calories. On the other hand, a man engaged in a very strenuous occupation may require perhaps up to 4000 calories. A common diet to use is a controlled carbohydrate diet utilising a system of 10 gram carbohydrate exchanges to give variety and allowing a free protein and fat intake.

Control of hyperglycaemia

For those patients in whom dietary measures are not successful, there are two main groups of drugs which control hyperglycaemia: (a) oral antidiabetic agents and (b) insulin.

Oral antidiabetic agents may be divided into the sulphonylureas and the biguanides. Of these the sulphonylureas are the most widely used. This group of drugs is considered to act by stimulating the beta cells of the pancreas to produce more insulin. They are, therefore, ineffective when there is exhaustion of the islet cell tissue as in the young ketotic insulin dependent diabetic patient. It is accepted that a contraindication to the use of these drugs is any evidence of ketosis, either at present or previously. Where one is considering changing from insulin to a sulphonylurea it is generally accepted that this is likely to be unsuccessful when the daily dose of insulin exceeds 40 units per day. Within the group of sulphonylureas there are several different drugs which all act by the same mechanism, the main difference being the duration of action and the potency. Of these drugs probably the most widely used in the United Kingdom is chlorpropamide. This has the advantage of requiring only a once daily treatment regime. The duration of action of this particular preparation is approximately 36 hours. The usual starting dose is between 125 and 250 mg daily half an hour before breakfast. In elderly people one must watch carefully for any signs of nocturnal hypoglycaemia or of hypoglycaemic symptoms in the early morning before the next dose is due. Tolbutamide is a shorter acting oral sulphonylurea and requires to be given in a dose of 0·5 to 1 g 2 or 3 times per day. This drug is not now much used especially since it was the sulphonylurea which was suggested in studies in America to result in an increased incidence of ischaemic heart disease in treated patients. A recent addition to drugs of this group is glibenclamide which is the most potent, being used in doses of 2·5 to 5 mg once or twice per day. Its duration of action is intermediate between that of chlorpropamide and tolbutamide. Its potency is such that it can be used in some patients not fully controlled by chlorpropamide. Other similar new sulphonylurea drugs are on the market.

The other main group of oral antidiabetic agents is the biguanides and the two drugs used in clinical practice are metformin and phenformin. Both have a similar mode of action which is different from that of the sulphonylureas. They appear to have a hypoglycaemic action mainly through an insulin-like effect of increasing peripheral uptake of glucose into the tissues and do not appear to affect the synthesis or release of insulin. They have one advantage over the sulphonylureas in that they tend, when given to obese patients, to cause weight loss as opposed to the weight gain which is often seen when sulphonylureas are used without a strict dietary regime at the same time. The common side effect from the biguanides is gastrointestinal upset but occasionally with phenformin severe and sometimes fatal lactic acidosis may be found. This has caused metformin to be the preferred drug as it is very rarely associated with this complication. Metformin may however be associated with vitamin B_{12} deficiency.

In some patients who have not responded to sulphonylurea drugs in adequate dosage it may be possible to achieve control by giving a combination of a sulphonylurea with a biguanide but with glibenclamide the need for this has lessened. Usually, however, patients with difficulty in achieving control are best treated with insulin.

Insulin treatment is required where a diabetic patient either is not suitable for or does not respond to treatment with diet alone or with the diet coupled with an oral hypoglycaemic agent. A variety of different types of insulin is available. The insulins formerly commonly used were of beef origin but recently porcine insulins have become available and are useful in the occasional patient who develops a sensitivity to the beef insulin. Insulin of porcine origin is more like human insulin than is beef insulin and therefore causes fewer immunological problems. Since insulin is a protein hormone it requires to be given by injection and it is essential that the patient learns the management of his own injection technique and also is taught how to adjust the dose of insulin for intercurrent infection or other transient upsets.

The choice of preparation of insulin depends on the severity of the patient's clinical diabetic problem, the type of dosage required and the preference of the physician. Insulins can be divided into short-acting, medium-acting and long-acting insulins (Fig. 7.1). The suffix RI used to describe insulins, which stands for 'rarely immunogenic', has the same significance as MC (monocomponent) and indicates highly purified insulins.

In addition to the insulins shown in Table 7.1 there are proprietary mixtures of highly purified insulins available. Examples of these are 'Rapitard MC' which is a mixture of 25 per cent MC porcine insulin and 75 per cent MC crystalline bovine insulin, and 'Lentard MC' which is a mixture of 30 per cent amorphous MC porcine insulin and 70 per cent crystalline bovine insulin. These insulins are intended for once daily use but may require addition of a short acting MC insulin such as 'Actrapid' for increased early effect.

Highly purified forms of beef insulins are now coming on the market.

Table 7.1

Duration of Action	Traditional Insulins (Beef)	More Recently Developed Insulins (Beef)	Highly Purified ('Monocomponent') Insulins (Mainly porcine)
Short	Soluble Insulin	Neutral Insulin — 'Nuso'	Neutral Insulin (MC) —'Actrapid' 'Leo Neutral RI'
Medium	Isophane Insulin Globin Insulin (Rarely used)	Insulin Zinc Suspension (Amorphous) — 'Semilente'	Insulin Zinc Suspension (Amorphous) MC — 'Semitard' 'Leo Retard RI'
Long	Protamine Zinc Insulin (PZI)	Insulin Zinc Suspension — 'Lente' Insulin Zinc Suspension (Crystalline) — 'Ultralente'	Insulin Zinc Suspension (MC) —'Monotard' 'Novo Ultratard'

The standard short-acting insulin is soluble insulin (referred to as regular insulin in North America). This, or one of the more purified short acting insulins, is the insulin of choice to be used in treating an acute diabetic problem such as diabetic ketoacidosis or in relation to acute infections or a rapidly changing clinical situation such as an operative procedure. In these clinical situations it is usually given by the intravenous route, either by an infusion pump as outlined under the treatment of ketoacidosis or where the problem is less acute by the addition of small doses of insulin such as 10 units/litre to an intravenous infusion of dextrose.

Soluble insulin is not normally used as a long term treatment of diabetes mellitus in the majority of patients. There are, however, some patients whose diabetes is unstable or whose occupation makes it difficult to obtain regular meal times and these patients may be best managed on two or more doses of subcutaneous soluble insulin per day as opposed to any attempt to put them on a single daily injection of insulin.

Of the medium- to long-acting insulins the one which has probably been most used in the United Kingdom is lente insulin. This is a mixture of two other insulins, one short-acting and one long-acting, referred to as semilente and ultralente respectively. Many diabetic patients can be stabilised on one single daily dose of lente insulin. In a new diabetic patient of only moderate severity it would be reasonable to start treatment with a dose of around 20 units of lente insulin daily and adjust this up or down as required by 4 units per day. In general if a patient requires more than 60 units of lente insulin daily he is not likely to be well controlled in the long term on this preparation and arrangements should be made to change his regime to one of the other insulins. Isophane insulin and globin insulin (now rarely used) are other insulins with a medium duration of action. Isophane insulin (insulin coupled to protamine) used with soluble insulin as twice daily injections is a popular regime.

The classical long-acting insulin is protamine zinc insulin (PZI) in which the insulin is coupled to protamine and zinc in an attempt to delay its breakdown. It is only the exceptional diabetic patient who can be adequately controlled on a single dose of protamine zinc insulin alone. Most patients in whom this particular preparation is used require an additional short-acting insulin preparation. This is usually given in the form of soluble insulin. It is important that the patient who is taking both soluble insulin and PZI appreciates that he must not mix them in the same syringe. The soluble insulin becomes converted to the long-acting preparation in these circumstances.

Recently, purified porcine insulins without the proinsulin contaminant ('monocomponent' insulin) have become available. These are manufactured in a range of preparations to give a variety of duration of action. When a patient is changed from one of the traditional insulins to a 'monocomponent' insulin usually a smaller dose is required. The supply of these insulins at present is not sufficient to treat every patient and so they have not completely displaced the more traditional insulins. They may offer advantages in the patient with insulin antibodies as the antibody production may be to the contaminants present in the traditional insulin. A more theoretical advantage is the possibility that use of these purified insulins might result in a lower incidence of diabetic complications. This will require long term trials to verify.

Complications of insulin therapy. These can be divided into local and general.

Local complications include such obvious things as infection at the site of injection due to faulty sterilisation technique. Sometimes more specific abnormalities such as localised atrophy or local hypertrophy of the subcutaneous fat at the site of injection may be seen. There is recent evidence that this atrophy is due to impurities in the older insulins and that use of the 'monocomponent' insulins will not only avoid this complication but will reverse fat atrophy when injected into the affected site.

Of the general reactions the most important is of course hypoglycaemia due to excessive insulin dosage. This is dealt with under the heading of hypoglycaemic coma. Apart from this the systemic effects of insulin therapy are few. The occasional patient develops hypersensitivity to insulin and may develop an urticarial rash. Many of these patients can be managed by a change from beef to porcine insulin.

In the occasional patient resistance to insulin therapy may develop due to the development of specific insulin antibodies. This may require the use of dosage of insulin of several hundred units per day. Sometimes the use of steroids will help to diminish this problem by diminishing the tendency to form insulin antibodies. This is the one situation where steroids may improve diabetic control. Usually the administration of glucocorticoid drugs to a diabetic patient results in deterioration of the diabetic state. The 'monocomponent' insulins are of value in this situation and have greatly reduced the problem of management of patients with insulin resistance.

Diabetic ketoacidosis

This is the most important emergency complication of diabetes mellitus and is a major cause of mortality in such patients. The history often is obtained that the patient has had a bowel upset or a cold or influenza-like illness, has stopped eating, stopped taking his insulin, and over two or three days has become progressively drowsy, developed laboured breathing and eventually lapsed into a state of semi- or complete unconsciousness. In some patients this condition may be the initial presenting feature of the diabetic state.

On examination these patients are severely dehydrated with marked loss of skin turgor. The smell of ketones in the patient's breath is very obvious even on just entering the sickroom and hyperventilation will be obvious (Kussmaul respiration). In some patients with diabetic ketoacidosis, abdominal pain may be so severe as to mimic an acute intra-abdominal crisis. This symptom can cause confusion if the patient is not known to be a diabetic and the situation is further complicated by the fact that the condition of diabetic ketoacidosis is often precipitated by intercurrent bowel upsets. Vomiting is a frequent clinical feature of diabetic ketoacidosis and most patients benefit from having their gastric contents aspirated by nasogastric tube.

Biochemical examination of the blood reveals blood sugar values of 25 mmol/l and upwards associated with a severe degree of acidosis with a pH sometimes below 7. The urine contains much sugar and ketones.

It is obvious that the important elements of treatment are:

1. Rehydration
2. Cure of the hyperglycaemia
3. Cure of the acidosis
4. Treatment of any precipitating infection.

As regards the first, the important thing is to give an adequate amount of fluid. This is usually given in the form of 0·9 per cent saline. The amount of fluid required may be very large. It is customary to give at least a litre by rapid infusion and then a litre every one to two hours until the dehydration is corrected. Dextrose should not be used initially as the patient is already hyperglycaemic. Since changes in blood sugar are used to monitor treatment these would be obscured by giving dextrose infusions.

The hyperglycaemia is corrected by giving insulin in the form of soluble insulin. There are various regimes which have been used and in the past it has been customary to use very large doses of insulin either by intravenous or combined intravenous and subcutaneous injection. This could involve the administration of several hundred units of insulin over the course of the first day of treatment. Recently it has been shown that much smaller doses of insulin can achieve adequate clinical and biochemical control when given by either the intramuscular or the intravenous route and satisfactory control can be achieved by intravenous infusion of the order of 5 units of soluble insulin per hour preferably by a constant rate infusion pump.

There is some controversy about correction of the acidosis. In general, provided the patient is given adequate fluid and adequate insulin the acidosis gradually corrects itself as the patient's biochemical state readjusts. Formerly there was a vogue for treating the acidosis actively by giving large amounts of bicarbonate or lactate intravenously. It is now recognised that the blood lactate level is elevated in diabetic ketoacidosis and it is not recommended that additional lactate be given. If one is giving treatment with bicarbonate one should not aim for full correction of the acidosis to an 'ideal' biochemical state because there is a danger of making the patient alkalotic. The administration of bicarbonate also aggravates the tendency to hypokalaemia (see below).

Another important aspect of treatment of diabetes is proper correction of electrolyte balance and in this respect potassium is the ion which is of major interest. As glucose moves from the plasma into the cell under the influence of insulin it takes with it substantial amounts of potassium from the plasma and although many of these patients with ketoacidosis have a normal or even on occasions a high serum potassium on admission this will usually rapidly fall with adequate correction of the dehydration and hyperglycaemia. It is therefore important to monitor the potassium regularly and to give supplementary intravenous potassium, as required.

Once the patient is rehydrated and the hyperglycaemia is under control the intravenous infusion is usually changed to one of dextrose and the patient is then managed on a regime of soluble or other short acting insulin given subcutaneously 8-hourly according to monitoring of the blood sugar values. Most of these patients recover rapidly unless there is any intercurrent disease and usually are able to resume a liquid diet the following day and then rapidly get back to their normal diet and insulin therapy. If any site of infection is found this must be treated vigorously by appropriate antibiotic therapy.

Hyperosmolar diabetic coma

This is a recently described entity in which usually elderly patients, who often are mild diabetics or even in whom there is no preceding evidence of diabetes, develop a state of deep unconsciousness. On examination such patients are dehydrated but not ketotic. The striking finding biochemically is the degree of hyperosmolality present in the serum, blood sugar values often being greater than 55 mmol/l. The prognosis of this condition is poor and indeed many of these patients appear to have their condition precipitated by intercurrent illness such as strokes which will affect the prognosis adversely. The treatment of these patients is controversial. The usual fluid replacement given is half strength saline and the hyperglycaemia is controlled by insulin as already outlined for ketoacidosis. Of those patients who do recover from this life-threatening situation many appear not to require any long term antidiabetic treatment.

Treatment of the chronic complications of diabetes mellitus

It will be recalled that the three important long term complications of diabetes mellitus are neuropathy, nephropathy and ophthalmopathy. It must be remembered that when one of the triad of complications is present usually it will be found that at least one of the others is also present.

What is not yet clear, even after many years study, is whether or not the development and the progression of these lesions is necessarily dependent on the adequacy or otherwise of diabetic control. There may be factors of which we are not yet aware which determine the progression of the disease in each individual.

As already mentioned, there is some evidence that in the early stages the neuropathy of diabetes mellitus may be reversible by good diabetic control implying that this is a metabolic disorder. When, however, a chronic neuropathy is established there is no good evidence that this is reversible by diabetic control. Fortunately, in many patients the degree of disability is far less than might be suggested from the signs elicited on neurological examination.

Once the renal lesion of diabetes mellitus is established there is no known treatment which influences the progression of the illness. The management of this problem is obviously that of chronic renal failure of any type with appropriate dietary restriction of protein. This obviously poses a problem for a patient who already has dietary restriction of carbohydrate because of his diabetes mellitus.

The ophthalmopathy of diabetes mellitus usually is not troublesome unless it directly affects the macular region or causes retinitis proliferans. There have been claims made for the maintenance of severe degrees of retinopathy being dependent on anterior pituitary function. It has been suggested that ablation of the anterior pituitary by surgery, stalk section or other techniques may arrest or indeed reverse the process. There is no firm evidence that this is indeed so. Potentially, if, as has been suggested, growth hormone is one of the important causal factors it may be that growth hormone release inhibitory factor, somatostatin, may come in the future to have a useful place in treatment of this condition. In selected patients benefit may be obtained by causing areas of photocoagulation of the retina. The selection of these patients is a matter of expert ophthalmological management.

Cataracts in the diabetic patient should be dealt with in their own right when an appropriate degree of maturity has been reached to allow ophthalmic surgery.

The other complications such as peripheral vascular disease must be dealt with in their own right. Often they may require local amputation but in this respect the diabetic patient is often able to have a more peripheral amputation than would be feasible in the patient with pure atherosclerotic disease of the same degree. This is because part of the problem of the diabetic patient is due to the accompanying neuropathy rather than entirely to vascular disease.

ATTEMPTS TO ACHIEVE IDEAL DIABETIC CONTROL

Recently various attempts have been made to achieve ideal diabetic control especially during pregnancy, or in the treatment of unstable 'brittle' diabetes. This has been approached by various methods such as

a) Self monitoring of blood glucose. The patient carries out blood glucose profiles on blood obtained by finger prick onto special filter papers and using a commercially available direct reading glucose meter. The dose of insulin required can be adjusted daily by the patient.

b) Continuous subcutaneous infusion of insulin over a period of weeks to months using a small infusion pump and a subcutaneous canula. In some systems the patient can give a boosting dose of insulin before meals in addition to the constant infusion.

c) The artificial pancreas in which there is continuous sampling of blood sugar and immediate computerised control of an intravenous infusion of insulin in response to the result. At present this is a cumbersome system only suitable for short term use.

d) Pancreatic transplantation or intravenous injection of isolated islets has been used but both of these techniques are in the experimental stage.

Of these techniques, self monitoring of blood glucose holds out the greatest promise of wide applicability.

PRACTICAL POINTS IN THE MANAGEMENT OF DIABETES MELLITUS

It is very important that the patient should fully understand his disease and his treatment insofar as his intelligence will allow. He must be carefully instructed in dosage of insulin and in the technique of injection and sterilisation of the syringe and needles. As regards the dosage of insulin this sometimes causes confusion because of the different strengths in which insulin is marketed. Most insulins are marketed in 40 and 80 units/ml strength with the exception of soluble (regular) insulin which is marketed in the strength of 20 units/ml, in addition to the 40 and 80 strength. In many clinics the patient is instructed not in terms of units of insulin but in terms of marks on his syringe. To determine the dose of insulin, if one knows the number of marks on the syringe and the strength the patient is taking, the dose is simply worked out by multiplying the number of marks by 2 when the patient is taking 40 units/ml and by 4 if he is taking 80 units/ml strength.

In recent years especially in North America an attempt has been made to simplify insulin administration by using a single strength insulin of 100 units/ml in conjunction with an insulin syringe graduated in 100 marks to 1 ml. This logical development is likely to be introduced in the U.K. in the near future.

The patient must understand the importance of proper urine testing and should be instructed to empty his bladder 20–30 minutes before collecting the sample to be tested. If this precaution is not observed, he may be making judgements on urine passed some hours previously.

It is important that the diabetic patient should take great care of his personal hygiene. It is particularly important that he takes great care of his feet and if necessary attends a qualified chiropodist regularly to try and avoid any damage to the skin which might be the initial source of gangrene.

Hypoglycaemic states

1. *Insulin overdosage*

There are many listed conditions which cause hypoglycaemia but much the most important of these in clinical practice is the excessive administration of insulin. Students often are confused about the differential diagnosis of hypoglycaemic coma from a hyperglycaemic coma but in clinical practice the diagnosis is not difficult especially if a good history is obtained and the patient is known to be a diabetic. The patient who develops a hypoglycaemic coma does so rapidly in contrast to the 2 or 3 days in which a hyperglycaemic coma develops. The patient in a hypoglycaemic coma is not dehydrated and is not acidotic. Instead he has a fast bounding pulse and is usually sweating and looks pale. These features are all manifestations of the adrenaline response which is attempting to raise the blood sugar by causing glycogenolysis. Characteristically on examination of the hypoglycaemic patient the striking feature is bilateral extensor plantar responses which revert when a normal blood sugar level is resumed.

Sometimes, however, if there is no adequate history there may be confusion between a hypoglycaemic and a hyperglycaemic coma. The correct practical thing to do is to take off a blood sample for later testing for glucose and to give through the same needle an intravenous injection of 50 per cent glucose. This will do no harm if the patient is in hyperglycaemic coma and will cure the condition if the patient is in hypoglycaemic coma. An alternative to giving intravenous glucose is to administer glucagon subcutaneously. This is, however, less certain of action as it requires a store of liver glycogen to be present to have an effective response. It is very important that hypoglycaemic coma is adequately and rapidly treated because if this is not done the patient may suffer permanent brain damage. On occasion one may encounter self-administration of insulin in mentally disturbed patients who have access to the drug and the author has seen one extreme example where a hospital porter administered to himself 6000 units of soluble insulin in a suicidal bid. This was successful despite the infusion of massive amounts of glucose because some hours elapsed before he was brought for medical attention.

Sometimes in patients receiving long-acting insulin preparations such as PZI or long-acting oral hypoglycaemic drugs such as chlorpropamide, the manifestations of hypoglycaemic coma may be much more subtle. The patient is often elderly, may merely complain of a headache when wakening in the morning and may appear slightly confused, a symptom which is often attributed to cerebral atherosclerosis. It may be found, however, that these patients are hypoglycaemic and of course it is very important to deal with this by reducing the dose of hypoglycaemic therapy or discontinuing this where possible.

2. *Insulinoma*

Other causes of hypoglycaemia are rare in clinical practice. One of the best known is hypoglycaemia due to a spontaneous insulin secreting tumour (insulinoma). This is a tumour of the beta cells of the pancreatic islets and the patient may present in a sudden hypoglycaemic coma which resembles that found after insulin administration. However, the condition may be manifest in a more neuropsychiatric way, for instance by bizarre behaviour or epileptiform seizures. It is therefore important to exclude hypoglycaemia in patients presenting with such conditions.

The first step in the differential diagnosis of these patients is to confirm that they are indeed hypoglycaemic. It is a truism that a patient cannot be in a hypoglycaemic coma unless he or she is hypoglycaemic. It is surprising how often this elementary fact is forgotten! For the diagnosis of insulinoma the patient should classically not only be biochemically hypoglycaemic but should have symptoms attributable to hypoglycaemia which are reversible with glucose administration. This spectrum of clinical features constitutes Whipple's triad.

If the patient is shown to be hypoglycaemic, the essential diagnostic feature of an insulinoma is the demonstration that at hypoglycaemic levels of blood sugar the patient still is secreting insulin. This is in contrast to the normal subject where when the blood sugar falls to low levels release of insulin ceases. Therefore, the important diagnostic step is to collect three morning samples of blood for fasting glucose and insulin. If the insulin level is high and the patient is hypoglycaemic this very strongly suggests the presence of an insulinoma.

A convenient way to express this discrepancy between insulin and glucose is to use the amended insulin/glucose ratio which is expressed as

$$\frac{\text{Plasma insulin (mU/l)}}{\text{Plasma glucose (mmol/l)} - 1{\cdot}7}$$

The correction factor is because the plasma insulin is normally undetectable at a plasma glucose level of 1·7 mmol/l. Normal values for the amended insulin/glucose ratio are <10 and for patients with insulinomas >30.

If more detailed studies of the nature of the insulin secreted are performed it will be found that a significantly larger proportion of the insulin is present as proinsulin. Measurement of this fraction has been claimed to be of value as a test of insulinoma.

Previously attempts were made to stimulate the pancreas by giving an injection of tolbutamide intravenously. This drug stimulates the beta cells of the islet tissue and the resultant rise in the plasma insulin in normal patients causes hypoglycaemia which lasts about two hours. In some patients with an insulinoma, tolbutamide causes an excessive insulin response with a fall in blood sugar which takes longer to return to normal. This test is, however, not completely reliable. This also applies to the other stimulatory tests such as the glucagon test and the arginine infusion test.

One test which has been recently developed is the fish insulin test. The principle of this test is that the patient is made hypoglycaemic by giving fish insulin which is biologically effective in the human but which can be distinguished by radioimmunoassay from human insulin. At hypoglycaemic levels of plasma glucose, the patient's endogenous insulin release should be inhibited but in patients with an insulinoma this does not happen. It, therefore, is a form of 'insulinoma suppression test' rather than an 'insulinoma stimulation test' as with tolbutamide. In practice, although only comparatively small numbers of patients have been studied, it has given useful results.

Where the evidence points to the patient having an insulinoma an exploration of the abdomen should be undertaken. This operation is usually preceded by coeliac axis angiography and CAT scanning of the pancreas in an attempt to demonstrate and localise the tumour. One or sometimes more insulinomas can be found usually towards the tail of the pancreas. Where the biochemical evidence is strong but no discrete tumour can be found it is customary to resect approximately two-thirds of the pancreas, in the hope that a small adenoma is removed. It must be remembered that in some patients the tumour is malignant. In patients with hypoglycaemia in whom an insulinoma cannot be found or in patients with a malignant insulinoma which cannot be fully resected treatment can be given by using either diazoxide or streptozotocin. The former is a drug of the thiazide type used in the emergency treatment of hypertension. It has the effect of preventing insulin release from the beta cells of the pancreas. The latter drug is an antibiotic which has antimitotic properties.

3. *Early diabetes mellitus*

Paradoxically some patients with diabetes mellitus may initially present as cases of hypoglycaemia. These patients are usually the maturity onset type of diabetic patient in whom there is an excessive insulin response which is delayed and therefore out of phase with the rise in blood sugar. In such patients there may be times when the patient becomes hypoglycaemic and it has been suggested that such patients may be managed by giving a small dose of a sulphonylurea drug to stimulate an earlier release of insulin which hopefully will coincide with the sugar peak and thus remove the symptoms.

4. *Non-endocrine tumours*

In occasional patients hypoglycaemia may be associated with non-endocrine tumours. This is dealt with in the appropriate chapter.

5. *Miscellaneous causes of hypoglycaemia*

Other conditions such as severe liver disease may also be associated with hypoglycaemia especially following the ingestion of alcohol which inhibits the process of hepatic gluconeogenesis.

It should be noticed, however, that there are many patients who present with symptoms suggestive of hypoglycaemia in whom there is no good documentary evidence of hypoglycaemia. This often occurs in rather nervous patients in some of whom it appears that symptoms can indeed be warded off by taking extra sugar. This therapeutic response however does not itself constitute a diagnosis of hypoglycaemia as a cause of the patient's symptoms.

FURTHER READING

Alberti K G M M 1976 Disorders of carbohydrate metabolism excluding diabetes. Clinics in endocrinology and metabolism 5: 3

Bloom J, Ireland J 1980 A colour atlas of diabetes. Wolfe Medical Publications Ltd, London

Oakley W G, Pyke D A, Taylor K W 1978 Diabetes and its management, 3rd edn. Blackwell Scientific Publications, Oxford

Podolsky S 1978 Diabetes mellitus. Medical Clinics of North America 62: 4

Tattersall R 1977 Diabetes. Clinics in Endocrinology and Metabolism 6: 2

8

Parathyroid glands and metabolic bone disease

ANATOMY

The parathyroid glands are derived from the 3rd and 4th branchial pouches of the primitive fore-gut. These same structures are associated with development of the thyroid gland and for this reason it is not surprising that the parathyroid glands are usually situated in close proximity to the thyroid. The typical number of parathyroid glands in the human is 4, 2 usually situated in the region of the upper and 2 in the region of the lower pole of the thyroid, both pairs being situated on the posterior aspect of the thyroid. Indeed at times the parathyroid glands may appear at operation to be buried within the substance of the thyroid gland.

It is not, however, uncommon for a larger number of parathyroid glands to be present in the human. There may be as many as 10 in number. Although most are situated in the neck, some may be situated in widely dispersed situations such as the anterior mediastinum. This fact is important to bear in mind during parathyroid surgery which may require not only exploration of the neck but on occasion the much more formidable operation of opening the chest and inspecting the anterior mediastinal contents.

When examined microscopically the parathyroid glands are seen to be made up of three main types of cells, (1) small darkly staining cells—the chief cells; (2) cells which stain with eosin—the oxyphil or eosinophil cells, and (3) large clear cells referred to as water-clear cells. These latter two types of cell appear to be derived from the chief cells and seem to be potentially capable of secreting parathyroid hormone.

THE PHYSIOLOGICAL ROLE OF PARATHORMONE

The important role of parathormone in normal physiology seems to be to maintain the level of plasma calcium and this it does by mobilising calcium from bone, increasing calcium resorption from the gut and increasing calcium reabsorption from the renal tubules. Parathormone secretion appears to control specifically the level of the ionised serum calcium. This distinction is important because in normal conditions approximately half the serum calcium is bound to albumin and half is ionised. A further smaller fraction is complexed with organic ions. It appears that the ionised form of calcium is the important one physiologically and it is on the concentration of this part of the serum calcium that the control of parathyroid hormone secretion hinges. In conditions where the ionised serum calcium falls, the parathyroid gland is stimulated to secrete parathormone in order to raise it. Conversely when the serum calcium rises, under normal conditions the secretion of parathormone is removed giving a fine control of the level of serum calcium by a negative feedback mechanism. The parathyroid gland does not appear to be under any direct control from the pituitary gland although growth hormone seems to have some stimulatory effect on parathyroid function. This, however, is not nearly as important as the controlling effect of serum ionised calcium.

Until recently it was believed that the control of the serum calcium depended entirely on the negative feedback control of parathyroid function. More recently it has been realised that in the human, as in other animals, there is a calcium lowering hormone, calcitonin, which is produced from the 'C' cells of the thyroid gland and whose function appears to be to lower the serum calcium by preventing resorption of bone. This hormone is dealt with in detail in the chapter on the thyroid gland. Calcitonin therefore acts as a further regulator of the serum calcium level by antagonising the effect of parathormone on the resorption of calcium from bone.

Apart from its effect on the serum calcium, parathormone has an effect on phosphate metabolism by causing loss of phosphate from the renal tubules by lowering the tubular transport maximum for phosphate (T_mP) with resulting phosphaturia. Indeed it is believed by some authorities that phosphate leak from the kidney is the most important effect physiologically and that the effects of parathormone on calcium resorption from the gut and from bone are secondary to the phosphaturia.

ROLE OF VITAMIN D IN CALCIUM HOMEOSTASIS

Although not strictly speaking a hormone, vitamin D has such important effects on calcium homeostasis that it is essential to consider its role in calcium metabolism. It was recognised early on from the pioneering work of Mellanby that vitamin D was essential in prevention of rickets in puppies. It thus appeared to be an essential food factor and to fulfil the role required by the term vitamin. There was some initial controversy when it was shown that rickets could be prevented by exposure to sunlight, either natural or artificial. The conflict between these two opposing views was resolved when it was shown that the effect of ultraviolet light was to cause the conversion of precursor sterols to vitamin D. In animals this occurs in the skin. There is a variety of vitamin D-like sterols. Vitamin D_2 (calciferol) is of plant origin. The usual form found in animal products is vitamin D_3 (cholecalciferol). This is a fat soluble vitamin which is contained in natural dairy produce or is artifically added to such things as margarine or infant foods (Fig. 8.1).

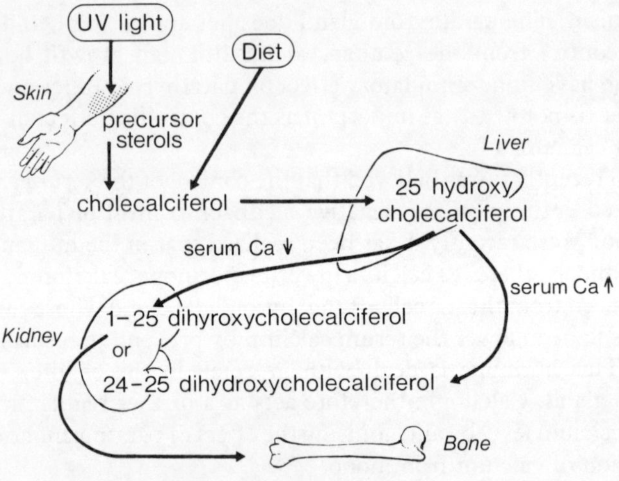

Fig. 8.1 Pathways of vitamin D metabolism

The main action of vitamin D appears to be to promote the absorption of calcium from the gut. It also however promotes the resorption of calcium and phosphorus from bone. Its actions are, therefore, complex and in some senses antagonistic although the net effect is usually to promote calcium retention, because of the over-riding effect of the vitamin on the gut.

Recent work has shown that the metabolism of vitamin D is much more complex than had been previously thought. It had been recognised for some time that cholecalciferol was converted in the liver to another compound 25-hydroxycholecalciferol. This was more active in preventing rickets than the parent compound. More recently it has been shown that the kidney is also important in the control of vitamin D metabolism by its action in further converting the

25-hydroxycholecalciferol to one of two other forms, namely 24,25-dihydroxycholecalciferol and 1,25-dihydroxycholecalciferol. This latter compound is an extremely potent derivative of vitamin D whereas the 24,25-dihydroxycholecalciferol is not nearly so potent. It appears that the 1-alpha-hydroxylation step is very important biologically because synthetic compounds such as 1-alpha-hydroxycholecalciferol are extremely potent in man. It would appear that in normal circumstances the kidney preferentially manufactures 24,25-dihydroxycholecalciferol but under conditions of low serum ionised calcium, low serum or intracellular phosphate and raised levels of parathyroid hormone, growth hormone, prolactin and placental lactogen, there is preferential secretion of 1,25-dihydroxycholecalciferol. In this way the kidney exerts a further fine control on calcium homeostasis. In this respect the kidney is acting as an endocrine organ in addition to its usual excretory function. It will be remembered that this is not the only endocrine effect of the kidney because the kidney also is responsible for secreting renin which controls the angiotensin/sodium control mechanism and erythropoetin which stimulates red cell synthesis. The kidney, therefore, would seem to be yet another organ which has a dual function, being partly endocrine and partly excretory.

CALCIUM KINETICS

It will therefore be seen that the control of calcium metabolism is extremely complex. On one hand parathormone stimulates the absorption of calcium from the gut but also mobilises calcium from the bone. Calcitonin acts to diminish the serum calcium level by preventing resorption of calcium from bone. This however is only of importance where bone turnover is high. Vitamin D increases the absorption of calcium from the gut but also mobilises calcium from bone.

It is clear, therefore, that this is a very dynamic situation and it is wrong to look upon the calcium stores in bone as static. There are constant metabolic shifts of calcium between the bone, the plasma, the extracellular fluid, the kidney and the gut. Since bone is much the largest store of calcium in the body obviously the state of the calcium content of bone is one further factor determining the serum calcium level. Attempts have been made by isotopic studies to look at each particular part of the control of calcium metabolism in the human but there is so much interplay between the various factors involved that it is obviously very difficult, if not impossible, to give absolute values to the calcium shifts between one compartment and another.

STRUCTURE OF NORMAL BONE

From the point of view of the embryologist there are two distinct types of bone in the human, (a) cartilaginous bone where initially in fetal life there is a cartilaginous structure laid down which is later invaded by osteoblasts to give rise to bone by transforming the cartilage into ossified material and (b) membranous bone where a layer of fibrous tissue is laid down which later becomes ossified and changed into bone without having passed through a cartilaginous stage. Broadly speaking the flat bones such as the skull, facial bones and sternum arise from membranous bone whereas the rest of the bones including all the limb bones arise from cartilaginous bone.

Microscopically bone is composed of concentric layers of calcified material which consist of crystals of hydroxyapatite laid down in a regular lamellar pattern on a protein matrix. Bones are of course not uniform throughout their diameter or length. Typically in the long bones there is an outer cylinder of compact bone with a marrow cavity. In the flat bones, such as the spine, the pelvic bones and iliac crest, the arrangement is an outer dense layer and a middle layer filled with a much more spongy arrangement of bone where the individual trabeculae can be seen.

In normal circumstances there is a good balance between the amount of protein matrix, which is largely formed of collagen, and the amount of calcification. When one looks at bone microscopically there usually is only a small area partially covering the bony trabeculae in which there is an excess of bone matrix which has not yet become calcified. The area of active calcification is usually denoted by a more densely staining area referred to as the calcification front. In abnormal conditions the amount of uncalcified bone matrix can be increased and there may be no obvious stainable calcification front.

Hormones involved in the control of bone formation

In addition to the hormones already mentioned namely parathormone, calcitonin and vitamin D and its metabolites many other hormones are involved in bone formation. The obvious one of these is growth hormone which as its name suggests is a major factor involved in growth of the skeleton. Growth hormone does not appear to be active itself directly on bone but it appears to influence the liver to manufacture another plasma factor, somatomedin ('sulphation factor') whose action is measured by its ability to increase the incorporation of sulphate into cartilage. By means of promoting the production of somatomedin, growth hormone increases the growth of cartilage which is later calcified.

Thyroid hormone is also important as can be seen readily in thyroid hormone deficient children where stunting of growth is regularly found and where there is a delay in bone development and in calcification. The thyroid hormones therefore like growth hormone have an anabolic effect on bone.

The other important anabolic hormones are the sex hormones which in the male is testosterone and in the female oestrogen. Both these hormones promote bone growth and development and both will accelerate epiphyseal closure if given in excess.

The most important catabolic hormones with regard to bone are hydrocortisone and other glucocorticoids. These act to break down bone by removing the bone matrix with secondary loss of the hydroxyapatite component. They also interfere with calcium absorption from the gut.

Tests of bone resorption and formation

In view of the various factors already discussed it is important to be able to get some measurement of bone formation and resorption. In the main this can be obtained by either biochemical, radiological or histological means.

1. *Biochemical*. Bone formation can be judged in clinical practice by assay of the alkaline phosphatase. This enzyme is produced by the osteoblasts in the bone and is subsequently excreted by the liver. The interpretation of a raised alkaline phosphatase level can therefore be complex and before attributing it to changes in bone one must make sure as far as possible that the patient's liver function is not abnormal. When in doubt it is possible to confirm whether the raised alkaline phosphatase level is of bone or hepatic origin by estimating the 5′-nucleotidase level. It should be noted that a raised alkaline phosphatase is often taken as an index of bone resorption but this is only valid insofar that usually when there is bone resorption there also is bone formation and therefore the alkaline phosphatase reflects both activities. As examples of its function in assessing bone formation it can be pointed out that the levels of serum alkaline phosphatase found at puberty are in excess of the adult range as are levels found with a healing fracture. Clearly in both instances the raised alkaline phosphatase is indicating bone formation and not bone resorption.

Bone resorptive disease is often first suggested by finding a raised calcium in association with a raised alkaline phosphatase. It should be noted, however, that neither of these is specific for bone resorption. A raised serum calcium is found in many diverse conditions. A raised alkaline phosphatase is, as stated above, often due to liver disease or increased bone formation. Perhaps the most specific test of bone destruction from the biochemical point of view is the plasma or urinary hydroxyproline level. Hydroxyproline is an aminoacid which exists almost entirely in collagen and since most of the bone protein matrix is made up of collagen the breakdown of this will result in increased levels of plasma and urinary hydroxyproline. Increased levels of hydroxyproline are also found in other endocrine diseases, notably in conditions where there is excess growth hormone or in thyrotoxicosis.

2. *Radiological.* In the growing child bone formation may be assessed by increased skeletal growth and increasing ossification, at the appropriate time, of the various epiphyseal centres. Thus the appearance of regular skeletal growth and a normal bone age as judged from one of the standard charts such as the Tanner-Whitehouse or the Greulich and Pyle atlas are good indicators of normal bone growth.

In the adult it is more difficult to assess bone formation and resorption but this has been attempted in various ways such as taking X-rays of the patient in a standard way and comparing the resulting film with previously prepared standards, usually in the form of an aluminium wedge of varying thickness. This technique is often applied to estimating the density of the bones in the spine. Other techniques are sometimes used for assessing the limb bones. A commonly used technique is a so-called metacarpal index. This is merely a mathematical expression of the amount of compact cortical bone to the total bone thickness in the mid point of the metacarpal bones. In general it is accepted that it is difficult to be precise by radiological techniques about minor degrees of bone loss and often as much as 25 per cent of the bone substance must be lost before the radiologist is prepared to report that there is decreased bone density. Yet another technique is to perform isotope densitometry. This is performed by passing a beam of γ-rays through a standard site, for example the forearm, and measuring the degree of absorption of the γ-rays by the bone.

3. *Histological.* Histological examination of bone obtained by percutaneous biopsy has the advantage of giving direct information on the degree of bone formation or resorption. This tissue, usually obtained from the iliac crest, allows some estimation of the amount of bone as judged from the ratio of the area of the trabeculae to the total area. Furthermore one can see whether or not there is an undue amount of non-calcified bone present and whether there is an active ossification process going on as judged by the presence or absence of a calcification front.

Tests of parathyroid function

These tests depend basically on biochemical studies of calcium, phosphate and alkaline phosphatase. For instance, when the parathyroid hormone is produced in excess the calcium level in the blood and in the urine is raised. This finding is usually coupled with a low serum inorganic phosphate and a high urinary phosphate because of the well known phosphaturic effect of parathormone. As a result of the parathyroid hormone's action there is active bone resorption and formation taking place. The alkaline phosphatase is therefore often raised when there is a considerable degree of bone involvement. Likewise the elevated levels of hydroxyproline in the plasma and in the urine reflect bone resorption.

Phosphate handling by the kidney has been expressed in many ways usually relating phosphate clearance to creatinine clearance. Changes in renal handling of phosphate do not bear a linear relationship to decreasing glomerular function as reflected by the creatinine clearance and the most valid index is to work out the tubular maximum reabsorption of phosphate and relate this to the glomerular filtration rate (T_mP/GFR). With a knowledge of plasma and urine phosphate and creatinine concentrations, this relationship may be calculated from a nomogram.

Conversely when parathormone production is lowered there is hypocalcaemia because of diminished ability to resorb calcium from the bone and to reabsorb calcium in the renal tubule. The serum inorganic phosphate will be high because of lack of parathormone effect on the renal tubules and the alkaline phosphatase is typically low. It can be shown that in hypoparathyroidism these changes can be reversed by the administration of parathormone (Ellsworth-Howard test). The basis of this classical test is to assess the effect of administered parathormone in altering the renal handling of phosphate. One would expect in a person with hypoparathyroidism that the administration of a potent parathormone preparation would cause increased excretion of phosphate. This is indeed what happens. At times, however, the changes in phosphate excretion may be difficult to interpret and where available the measurement of the excretion of cyclic AMP in the urine is preferable.

Parathyroid disease

Primary hyperparathyroidsim

In this condition there is an excess production of parathormone usually as the result of an adenoma of one or more parathyroid glands but sometimes this process results from the presence of a more diffuse hyperplastic process affecting all the parathyroid tissue. It has been recently recognised that primary chief cell hyperplasia may be associated with endocrine tumours affecting several glands such as adrenal, pituitary, thyroid and pancreas. On very rare occasions the condition can result from a malignant tumour of the parathyroid glands. The patient with primary hyperparathyroidism may present in a variety of ways. At least two of these are obvious from consideration of the effects of parathormone. Firstly, the patient may present because of renal stones. This results from the increased excretion of calcium in the urine as a result of the hypercalcaemia induced by parathormone. It is, therefore, essential that each patient presenting with renal stone should have a serum calcium measurement as a screening test to exclude hyperparathyroidism. In some patients with primary hyperparathyroidism, the calcium deposition may be in the substance of the renal tissue (nephrocalcinosis) rather than as renal stones.

It is perhaps worth noticing that many patients with renal stone in the absence of hyperparathyroidism appear to have hypercalciuria on the basis of hyperabsorption of calcium without having hypercalcaemia or any demonstrable upset of parathyroid function (idiopathic hypercalciuria).

Another type of patient with hyperparathyroidism presents primarily because of the bone problem. These patients may have painful bones, they may show evidence of a pathological fracture or develop a swelling over a bone as a result of an underlying bone cyst. Patients with multiple cystic lesions in their bones as a result of the process of primary hyperparathyroidism fall into the category of osteitis fibrosa cystica or von Recklinghausen's disease. It should be noted, however, that this is a rather uncommon and extreme degree of the condition in current medical practice and one would hope that the hyperparathyroidism would be diagnosed before this stage was reached.

Sometimes patients present with manifestations which are at first sight not obviously related to parathyroid malfunction. One of these which is well recognised is the presence of severe dyspepsia due to recurrent duodenal ulceration or pancreatitis and these are other clinical contexts in which it is worthwhile having the serum calcium assayed.

Patients may present because of symptoms of hypercalcaemia but often these are not obvious and usually the patient will only admit them on direct questioning. The typical symptoms of hypercalcaemia are polyuria, polydipsia, severe constipation, anorexia and vomiting. Although individually these symptoms are found in many conditions, as a combination of symptoms they are very strongly suggestive of hypercalcaemia. One additional feature is that many patients who have a significantly high serum calcium (as do patients with a low serum calcium) show symptoms of mental and emotional change. Such patients may be hyperkinetic to the point of being maniacal and often there is a gross impairment of memory. In some patients there may be striking redness of the conjunctivae due to calcium deposition. This can also be seen in the cornea by specialised techniques such as slit lamp examination.

One other relatively uncommon presentation of the condition is to the dental surgeon because of a tumour in the jaw, the so-called myeloid epulis. This is a tumour composed of osteoclastic tissue which presents as a soft tissue swelling in the region of the teeth.

Today, however, many patients diagnosed as hyperparathyroidism are being found in course of routine biochemical screening, especially when this is done by autoanalyser screening of blood. These patients may have minimal or even no symptoms.

Investigation. In any patient suspected of having hyperparathyroidism the first and most important test is an accurate determination of the serum calcium, preferably on more than one occasion. The normal range of serum calcium values is 2·2 to 2·6 mmol/l (conversion factor serum calcium in mmol/l × 4·008 = serum calcium in mg/100 ml). This test is ideally done in the fasting recumbent state and should be done without any venous occlusion being used. This is because eating, activity and venoconstriction all raise the serum calcium level and can introduce a critical error in a borderline case. Only on very few occasions will primary hyperparathyroidism be found in association with a normal serum calcium when estimated on several occasions. It is important that the level of the serum calcium is estimated in conjunction with an estimation of the plasma proteins because as previously explained approximately half of the serum calcium is protein bound and if for any reason the plasma proteins are low this will give an apparently low serum calcium value.

It is important to exclude other causes of hypercalcaemia. Common conditions are secondary carcinoma in bone, myelomatosis and vitamin D intoxication. Other causes which have been recognised but which are much less common are sarcoidosis, the milk-alkali syndrome, Addison's disease and thyrotoxicosis.

A test involving the administration of hydrocortisone has been used to eliminate some of these possibilities. Characteristically, patients with sarcoidosis, vitamin D intoxication and Addison's disease show a fall of serum calcium after steroid treatment (in the case of Addison's disease after replacement doses of glucocorticoids) but the response in the other conditions is variable. The diagnosis depends on their recognition from the history or examination.

In addition to estimating the serum calcium it is usual to estimate the serum inorganic phosphate, which one would expect to be low in hyperparathyroidism, and to estimate the alkaline phosphatase which may be high if bone involvement is marked. A normal serum inorganic phosphate in the adult is of the order of 0·8 to 1·5 mmol/l (conversion factor serum inorganic phosphate in mmol/l × 3·10=mg/100 ml).

Alterations in the serum inorganic phosphate are reflected in the urinary handling of phosphate and this should be confirmed by estimation of the TmP/GFR. It is customary to measure the urinary calcium which is usually elevated in the presence of hyperparathyroidism with hypercalcaemia. Characteristically the plasma chloride level is high since a condition of hyperchloraemic acidosis is present due to the effect of parathormone which causes renal loss of bicarbonate.

If at this point there is a convincingly elevated serum and urine calcium, a low inorganic phosphorus and a raised alkaline phosphatase, this is strong presumptive evidence that the patient has hyperparathyroidism.

It is then usual to carry out a skeletal survey. The classical radiological finding of hyperparathyroidism is evidence of bone resorption. This is often best seen on an X-ray of the hands where along the lateral margins of the middle phalanges striking evidence of bony resorption will often be seen. In addition, in the hands and in the long bones a varying degree of loss of bone density with, on occasions, multiple cystic formation may be seen in the bones. X-ray of the skull in severe cases shows a diffusely speckled pattern of calcification in the skull as a result of bone resorption and formation. Classically, provided the patient is not edentulous, an X-ray of the mandible and maxilla will show loss of the lamina dura which is a dense area of calcification round each tooth socket.

Having thus established that the patient almost certainly has excess parathormone production it might be thought obvious that one could confirm this by assay of parathormone in the serum. While this might be theoretically desirable, in fact estimation of serum parathormone plays little part in the routine diagnosis of the presence or absence of hyperparathyroidism. This is because often it is found that mild degrees of hyperparathyroidism do not cause significant elevation of the serum parathormone value in peripheral venous blood. Patients who have very obvious clinical and biochemical disease show raised parathormone levels but this is not helpful when the diagnosis is already so obvious. On some occasions, however, estimation of parathormone can be useful in localising parathyroid tissue (see below). Parathormone estimations also may be useful in the differential diagnosis of hypercalcaemia. In diseases other than hyperparathyroidism where hypercalcaemia is present, one would anticipate suppressed levels of parathormone. Only in hyperparathyroidism would one have the combination of a raised serum calcium and elevated serum parathormone value.

The next problem in diagnosis is to localise a possible parathyroid tumour. On rare occasions the tumour may be palpable but it is uncommon to feel the parathyroid tumour unless it is malignant. Sometimes an adenoma may cause indentation of the oesophagus and for this reason a barium swallow is sometimes a useful procedure. In recent years however there has been an attempt to try and localise parathyroid tissue by estimation of the parathormone content of blood obtained from different sites in the innominate, internal jugular and thyroid veins. Although, as stated above, estimation of the levels of parathormone in the systemic blood is not very helpful in establishing a diagnosis, it can be useful to estimate it more precisely in relation to probable tumour sites and this method is likely to gain ground especially where an initial exploratory operation has failed to localise an adenoma. Alternative techniques of localisation of parathyroid tissue by isotope scanning using selenium-labelled methionine have not in practice been found useful in most centres. CAT scanning has been used to a small extent.

Treatment. When the patient has been convincingly shown to have evidence of hypercalcaemia due to hyperparathyroidism, arrangements should be made for exploration of the neck by an experienced surgeon. Where the patient has very gross bone disease it is useful to attempt to get some recalcification of the bones before operation and this is done by giving an active form of vitamin D. If this is not done the patient with severe bone disease may develop extremely severe hypocalcaemia with striking tetany once a parathyroid adenoma has been removed. At operation the surgeon will localise and remove any parathyroid tumours or in the case of a diffuse hyperplastic process will remove three of the four parathyroid glands. In the case of the uncommon parathyroid carcinoma an attempt should be made to dissect out as much of the tumour as is possible.

A period of hypocalcaemia following the operation should be managed by infusion of calcium gluconate or the oral administration of calcium and vitamin D depending on the severity of the hypocalcaemia. Gradually the patient's calcium balance should right itself as the bones become adequately recalcified, the bone cysts will heal and the patient should become asymptomatic. Those patients with renal stone may of course require treatment of this condition in its own right.

On some occasions the serum calcium level may be so high as to indicate the need for emergency treatment. Often the correction of dehydration by saline infusion is sufficient to lower significantly the serum calcium but in other cases treatment with infusions of phosphate or sulphate may be required. A recent alternative treatment is the use of injections of calcitonin. Large doses of prednisolone may also be of value.

It is important to remember that sometimes hyperparathyroidism may be only one manifestation of a multiple endocrine disease problem which may affect the adrenal, the pituitary, the thyroid and the pancreas in addition.

Secondary hyperparathyroidism

The name secondary hyperparathyroidism is given to the situation where there is clear evidence of a predisposing disease process, usually malabsorption or chronic renal failure or less commonly specific tubular defects such as renal tubular acidosis—all these conditions result in severe lack of calcium with resultant parathyroid overactivity. The type of secondary hyperparathyroidism due to chronic renal failure is usually referred to as renal osteodystrophy and is dealt with under that heading.

By definition then, secondary hyperparathyroidism is a compensatory state and the compensatory rise in serum calcium should not exceed normal limits implying that the normal negative feedback control of parathyroid function by the serum calcium is still in effect.

Clinically the diagnosis is usually made in the context of one of the above mentioned conditions where the patient is found biochemically to have a normal serum calcium, a normal or low serum inorganic phosphate and an elevated alkaline phosphatase. No treatment is required for the parathyroid problem per se. Obviously removal or amelioration of the primary disease process will result in the restoration of normal parathyroid function.

Tertiary hyperparathyroidism

This term is applied where there is clear evidence that the patient has one of the predisposing conditions mentioned under secondary hyperparathyroidism but has passed through the phase of normal feedback control of parathyroid function to autonomous overactivity of parathyroid function. Classically this was thought to be due to the formation of an adenoma in hyperplastic tissue as a result of chronic hyperstimulation. It seems likely however that the sheer mass of hyperplastic tissue may predispose to a degree of autonomy and in some sense, an inappropriate degree of overactivity. In these patients, therefore, there is the biochemical picture of primary hyperparathyroidism with an elevated serum calcium, a low serum inorganic phosphate and an elevated alkaline phosphatase. The distinction between tertiary and primary hyperparathyroidism depends on the clear demonstration of an underlying condition predisposing to secondary hyperparathyroidism and the demonstration that the patient has indeed passed through a phase of normally compensated parathyroid function.

In tertiary hyperparathyroidism, in addition to treatment for the underlying disease process the patient requires treatment as in primary hyperparathyroidism. Removal of a parathyroid adenoma, if such can be demonstrated or of a major part of the hyperplastic glands, will result in lowering of the serum calcium to normal limits.

Hypoparathyroidism

In hypoparathyroidism the main clinical manifestations result from the low levels of the serum ionised calcium. The striking clinical result of this is increased neuromuscular excitability. This can be shown by the spontaneous onset of tetany or its production following the constriction of the blood supply to the arm by means of a sphygmomanometer cuff (Trousseau's sign). It can also become clinically demonstrated by stimulating the facial nerve by tapping over its course at the angle of the jaw. This results in twitching of the same side of the face, this sign being known as Chvostek's sign.

Tetany may also be seen in other conditions such as malabsorption which results in severe hypocalcaemia. It is not usually seen in chronic renal failure where the accompanying acidosis protects the patient by increasing the ionised fraction of calcium. Conversely, tetany may be seen with a normal serum calcium in alkalosis such as that caused by overbreathing.

In addition to these easily demonstrated effects on the peripheral nervous system there may be profound central nervous system effects such as depression. Moreover the patient with longstanding hypocalcaemia may develop cataracts and show skin changes with increased liability to fungal disease and brittleness of the nails.

The cause of hypoparathyroidism are:

1. Damage during thyroidectomy. This is by far the commonest cause of hypoparathyroidism. The incidence of parathyroid damage after thyroidectomy varies in different series depending on how closely it is looked for. It is generally accepted that around 5 per cent of patients show frank clinical hypoparathyroidism whereas up to 25 per cent may have evidence of impaired parathyroid reserve if more sophisticated testing such as EDTA infusion is adopted. It appears likely that the loss of parathyroid function following thyroidectomy

for thyrotoxicosis is not so much related to actual removal of the parathyroid glands, although this does sometimes happen especially where these are buried within the substance of the thyroid, as it is to damage to the parathyroids due to infarction of the glands from interference with their blood supply during dissection of the neck. Sometimes such damage appears to be temporary and the patient may recover normal function, presumably due to hypertrophy of the remaining tissue.

In some thyrotoxic patients, especially in those in whom the damage is temporary, it may be that one element in the development of apparent hypoparathyroidism is that the patient has had preceding severe calcium loss from the bones because of thyrotoxicosis and that following operation a great deal of calcium is removed from the plasma and extra cellular fluid to restore this deficit. Obviously in this circumstance, once the bones have been repleted with calcium the clinical problem of hypocalcaemic symptoms caused by a low serum calcium will resolve.

2. Idiopathic hypoparathyroidism. This is an uncommon condition where the patient spontaneously develops features of hypoparathyroidism. This may be manifest as spontaneous tetany or sometimes as actual convulsions. This latter symptom is important because phenobarbitone, which is often used in the treatment of convulsions, itself lowers the serum calcium by enzyme induction of vitamin D catabolising enzymes. The administration of phenobarbitone in this situation therefore may aggravate the clinical problem and the correct treatment for these hypocalcaemic convulsions is to cure the hypocalcaemia. Sometimes in addition patients may present to the ophthalmologist because of cataracts precipitated by calcium deposition in the lens. These patients may show what appears to be papilloedema together with seizures which, on investigation, is not due to any demonstrable space occupying lesion. The cause of the papilloedema in this condition is unknown but clearly the clinical picture may closely mimic brain tumour.

Patients with hypoparathyroidism are liable to an increased incidence of fungal infections of the skin and nails.

The condition of idiopathic hypoparathyroidism is to be distinguished from pseudohypoparathyroidism in which the patient typically shows the clinical features of stunting of growth, round face and has skeletal abnormalities, especially short metacarpal and metatarsal bones. They show the same biochemical abnormalities as in idiopathic hypoparathyroidism but do not respond to parathormone administration. It is now thought that pseudohypoparathyroidism represents end organ resistance to the effects of parathormone since it has been shown that the circulating parathormone values are usually elevated. The condition of pseudo-pseudohypoparathyroidism is where the somatic features of pseudohypoparathyroidism are associated with normal serum biochemical values. The distinction may be artificial since both pseudohypoparathyroidism and pseudo-pseudohypoparathyroidism may occur in one family and a patient diagnosed as pseudo-pseudo-hypoparathyroidism may later become hypocalcaemic.

Investigation of hypoparathyroidism. Apart from the clinical picture the essential feature is a low total and ionised serum calcium. There are of course many causes of a low serum calcium but in the main these are related to alteration of the plasma proteins or are due to severe malabsorption as in coeliac disease or advanced renal failure. Such conditions would be excluded during the course of routine investigations and demand treatment in their own right. The serum inorganic phosphate is typically elevated in hypoparathyroidism.

Some authors have emphasised the importance of stress tests such as EDTA infusion in the diagnosis of minor degrees of hypoparathyroidism in patients with normal serum calcium values. Symptoms such as tiredness and depression have been attributed to such subclinical 'deficiency' but it is by no means accepted that this is the case.

Radiological investigation may sometimes show the presence of subcutaneous calcification in patients with pseudohypoparathyroidism and X-ray of the skull may show the classical changes of calcification of the basal ganglia in both idiopathic and pseudohypoparathyroidism. Corneal calcification may be demonstrable by the ophthalmologist on slit lamp examination.

The common condition of post-thyroidectomy hypoparathyroidism will of course be diagnosed from the history in conjunction with the biochemical changes. To confirm the much less common condition of idiopathic hypoparathyroidism the response of the patient to the infusion of parathormone should be assessed (Ellsworth-Howard test). One would expect the patient with idiopathic hypoparathyroidism to show an excretion of phosphate and of cyclic AMP in the urine following the administration of this hormone. Typically pseudohypoparathyroidism is diagnosed when the patient has the same biochemical and clinical changes as idiopathic hypoparathyroidism but does not show a phosphaturic response to the administration of parathormone. It is likely that this distinction is rather artificial and there is evidence that the response to parathormone infusion may be dependent on the level of the serum calcium. Some patients who have been labelled as having pseudohypoparathyroidism appear to be capable of responding to parathormone once their serum calcium has been raised by appropriate therapy.

In some patients there is evidence that idiopathic hypoparathyroidism has an autoimmune basis. In these cases other autoimmune diseases such as Addison's disease or Hashimoto's thyroiditis may be found.

Treatment of hypoparathyroidism. The mainstay of treatment of hypoparathyroidism is the administration of vitamin D (cholecalciferol or one of its derivatives). These patients usually require large doses of vitamin D_3 of the order of 1·25 mg (50 000 units) or more daily. Better results have been claimed for various derivatives of vitamin D_3 such as dihydrotachysterol (AT 10), which is popular in the United States, and with the synthesis of more potent analogues such as 1-alpha-hydroxy vitamin D it may be possible to achieve more effective control. These patients require lifelong supervision and regular checks of the serum calcium to make sure that normal levels are reached but that excessive levels are not produced. One problem is that vitamin D, being a fat soluble vitamin, tends to have a long half-life as it is stored in the body fat and therefore following a build up of toxic amounts of Vitamin D, levels of serum calcium may remain elevated for up to 6 months. One clinical situation in which the dosage of vitamin D appears to vary is pregnancy and the puerperium and a particularly careful watch should be kept on the patient at this time.

In addition to vitamin D these patients may require calcium supplements and these are administered orally as effervescent tablets each containing 20 meq Ca^{++} along with vitamin D. In some patients supplements of magnesium are required in addition to calcium and vitamin D to fully correct the hypocalcaemia.

Metabolic bone disease

Osteoporosis

Osteoporosis is where there is proportional loss of bone matrix and calcium. It is one of the commonest bone diseases and indeed there are those who would claim that it is almost a physiological part of the ageing process. As already discussed, it is very difficult to judge minor degrees of calcium loss from bone. Even apparently sophisticated techniques such as X-rays of the bone compared against a standard aluminium step wedge or isotopic densitometry do not reveal minor changes. There is, however, no doubt that there is progressive loss of calcium from the bone with ageing. This starts to be significant at a much earlier age in the female than in the male and this change seems to take place about the time of the menopause. It will be remembered that in the female oestrogen is the most important anabolic hormone and is comparable with testosterone in the male in this respect. It would seem logical to attribute these changes to progressive diminution of ovarian production of oestrogen. The differential effect of bone loss between the sexes can be shown by the quite different fracture rates of such common sites as the neck of the femur or Colles' fracture. Further confirmation for this is that patients who have an early menopause by surgical removal or irradiation of the ovaries tend to develop osteoporosis at an earlier age than their more fortunate contemporaries who pass through a natural menopause at the usual time.

One possibility which has been raised is that patients who develop clinical problems with osteoporosis may have started with a smaller bone mass than those who do not. It has been argued that the defect in osteoporosis is not that the osteoporotic patient loses bone faster than a non-osteoporotic one but rather that the initial starting point is different. There is no definite evidence as to which of these arguments is correct.

In addition to the common clinical problem of 'physiological' osteoporosis of age, other endocrine diseases may be associated with increased tendency to osteoporosis. These include:

1. *Cushing's syndrome*. The osteoporosis is due to the catabolic effect of glucocorticoids on bone aggravated by impaired absorption of calcium from the gut.

2. *Thyrotoxicosis* causes increased bone turnover but with net loss of bone substance. Usually the patient who has thyrotoxicosis is diagnosed and treated before major bone problems have developed.

3. *Hypogonadism*. Both females with gonadal dysgenesis and males with hypogonadism who are not treated develop osteoporosis. This is easily explicable by the lack of anabolic hormones previously described.

In addition to such spontaneous endocrine disease the administration of large doses of glucocorticoids as long term therapy for rheumatoid arthritis or severe asthma will be associated with an increased tendency to osteoporosis.

Osteoporosis is seen also where there is immobility. It is obvious that movement in some ways strengthens the structure of bone. Osteoporosis which affects the bones adjacent to the joints is a regular feature of other disease processes such as rheumatoid arthritis. In part this may be due to the immobility induced by the arthritis.

We as yet do not know all the factors controlling the interchange of calcium between bone, extracellular fluid, plasma, kidney and gut and until we have a much clearer idea of the pathophysiology we will not be in a position to understand what ultimately causes loss of bone in osteoporosis.

Diagnosis of osteoporosis. The typical patient with osteoporosis is the middle-aged to elderly female who presents with backache, who has a marked kyphosis, the typical humped back of old age and who is found on radiological examination to have collapse of one or more of the thoracic vertebrae with biconcave deformities of the remaining vertebrae. In the introduction it was stressed that it is difficult to assess minor degrees of bone loss even using sophisticated techniques. Therefore the diagnosis of osteoporosis tends to be made by the radiologist when there has been already very gross loss of calcium from the bone, either when the patient is X-rayed for some incidental condition or much more commonly where the patient presents with a fracture. In these patients the biochemical tests are surprisingly normal. The serum calcium and inorganic phosphate are normal. The alkaline phosphatase may be temporarily elevated during the time a fracture is healing but is not otherwise abnormal. Histological examination of the bone shows that the bone is structurally normal although the trabeculae are thinner than is usually found. Osteoporosis, therefore, seems to be the result of the loss of calcium and bone matrix in proportional amounts. The remaining bone is not in any way abnormal except that the total quantity of it is less than usual.

Treatment of osteoporosis. 1. Treatment of the patient with established disease. The patient presenting with a typical fracture of the thoracic vertebrae and the patient presenting with a fracture of another site such as Colles' fracture are treated along conventional lines. The fractures heal adequately but with increasing deformity in the case of the fractures of the thoracic spine. The patient can be reassured that the backache is likely to ease. Such patients should be kept as mobile as possible, in view of the fact that immobility promotes bone loss.

Attempts have been made to reverse the process of osteoporosis. Approaches have been made along many lines such as administering calcium, sometimes in association with vitamin D, in the hope of correcting the negative calcium balance that exists. Active forms of Vitamin D such as 1α hydroxycholecalciferol are under trial on the basis that the ageing kidney might be defective in transforming 25–hydroxy vitamin D to the more active 1–25 dihydroxyvitamin D. Treatment with fluoride which is known to cause osteosclerosis when given in toxic amounts has also been tried either alone or in conjunction with vitamin D. Anabolic steroids, diphosphonates and oestrogens have also been used. Recently calcitonin has undergone clinical trials in this condition, but without convincing benefit.

With all these treatments there is no good evidence that there is a reversal of the osteoporotic process although they may prevent continuing bone loss. One of the reasons for the difficulty in assessing this type of treatment is that the techniques of assessing bone accretion are so poor that one would require a very dramatic increase in bone hydroxyapatite deposition before the current radiological or isotopic densitometric techniques would pick up the change. The efficiency of such treatments is, therefore, controversial.

2. Prevention of osteoporosis. This is a more attractive prospect in that there is hope that prevention might be much more effective than trying to treat established osteoporosis. For instance, in women who have had to have their ovaries removed at an early age it would seem reasonable to give supplemental oestrogens to prevent osteoporosis. Oestrogens have the added benefit of preventing dyspareunia due to atrophy of the sexual organs. It is not clear whether or not taking oestrogens from the time of the natural menopause is effective and therefore has a role in preventing osteoporosis.

Avoidance of the long term use of potent glucocorticoid drugs is another preventive measure. The question of whether increased physical activity throughout life would likewise be of help is unsettled as is the role of supplemental calcium or fluoride in the drinking water, which has also been proposed to prevent dental decay.

Osteomalacia

In contrast to osteoporosis, in osteomalacia there is a disproportionate loss of hydroxyapatite from the bones compared to loss of bone matrix. This is due to deficiency of calcium and vitamin D. Underlying causes of this lack of calcium and vitamin D may be a simple nutritional deficiency but usually this requires the patient to follow a very strict diet over a long time. On the other hand it may be the result of malabsorption, the cause of which may be iatrogenic, for example by previous gastric surgery, especially the operation of partial gastrectomy. It is not clear whether the newer gastric operations such as vagotomy and pyloroplasty are less troublesome with regard to osteomalacia. Alternatively there may be a renal condition such as renal tubular acidosis in which calcium is lost in large amounts in the urine. In addition to the loss of calcium, the lack of phosphate which favours bone mineralisation may be important.

Clinical presentation. The patient with osteomalacia tends to present not because of fractures but because of painful bones. In the early stages these pains may be poorly localised to bone. Since they are often associated with weakness of muscle they may be dismissed as some variety of soft tissue rheumatism and the true underlying disease may not be diagnosed. In more severe disease the muscles and the bones are very tender and proximal myopathy is so striking that the patient may walk with a waddling gait.

Diagnosis. The diagnosis of osteomalacia depends on a combination of biochemical and radiological findings.

There is a very typical biochemical picture in these patients. The calcium is usually low-normal or often frankly abnormally low, the serum inorganic phosphate is low (because of secondary hyperparathyroidism) and the alkaline phosphatase is raised for the same reason. Patients who present to the general physician or to the orthopaedic surgeon with bone pain ought therefore to have at least this degree of biochemical testing done as it will diagnose most patients with osteomalacia. In addition if the urinary calcium is measured it will be found to be low because of the inadequate absorption of calcium and/or vitamin D from the gut.

On radiological examination it will be found that there is loss of calcium from the bone. The hallmark which distinguishes osteomalacia radiologically from osteoporosis is the presence of areas of decalcification known as pseudofractures, Looser zones or Milkman fractures. These are areas of partial loss of bone continuity which occur over areas of stress, typical sites being the pubic rami, the upper part of the shaft and the neck of femur, and the lateral margin of the scapula. They can, however, occur in almost any site.

There is quite a different appearance on histological examination of a bone biopsy in osteomalacia from that found in osteoporosis. In osteomalacia the trabeculae are not thin as in osteoporosis. The striking feature is lack of calcification of the bone. The bony trabeculae are surrounded by large amounts of non-calcified bone matrix, the so-called osteoid tissue, and there is no active calcification front found on appropriate staining.

Treatment of osteomalacia. This consists of treating the underlying condition where possible but essentially the treatment is to give supplemental calcium and vitamin D. The dose used varies depending whether or not there is a significant degree of malabsorption. Obviously where the problem is simply one of dietary deficiency a relatively small dose of vitamin D_3 of the order of 0·125 mg (5000 units) per day will help to correct the deficiency whereas if there is a serious degree of malabsorption, large doses, even up to 1·25 mg (50 000 units), may on occasions be required. With this treatment there will be rapid resolution of the patient's bone pain and muscle weakness and restoration to normal health. Whether or not permanent replacement therapy is required depends on the circumstances of the particular patient such as whether the patient is able to alter her diet or whether there is some disease process present.

Rickets

This is the childhood counterpart of osteomalacia. It is a condition in which there is defective ossification of bone induced by a deficiency of vitamin D and/or calcium. It will be recalled that vitamin D is obtained usually from either dietary sources such as dairy produce or fortified margarine or alternatively from irradiation by sunlight of precursor sterols in the skin.

By far the commonest cause of rickets therefore is so-called nutritional rickets and this was an extremely common condition last century and earlier this century in the industrial cities of Britain due to a combination of inadequate diet and lack of adequate exposure to sunshine to compensate for this. When the aetiology of rickets was worked out in the 1920s and the opposing views that it could be cured by improving nutrition and also by exposure to ultraviolet light were reconciled rickets became virtually abolished in the United Kingdom. This was even so during the Second World War when careful attention was paid to the nutritional requirements of growing children. There has been recently a recrudescence of rickets amongst the Asian immigrant population in the United Kingdom. A great deal of work has been done on the aetiology of these cases of rickets. The condition is thought to be caused by a combination of factors, an Asiatic high cereal diet which has a high phytic content which binds the dietary calcium and prevents its absorption and may also contain antimineralising substances and the dark skin of the patient which may interfere with irradiation of the skin by the sun, which is of course much weaker in Britain than that to which they are accustomed.

Clinical presentation of rickets. Very gross rickets may present with obvious bowing of the legs, knock-knees, stunting of stature, broadening of the epiphyses at various sites, such as the wrists and over the costochondral junctions (the so-called rachitic rosary) and the deformed skull with frontal bossing. The residua of many of these features may be regularly seen in older members of the community in an industrial city such as Glasgow. In severe cases the degree of hypocalcaemia may be severe enough to cause tetany with laryngeal spasms and even convulsions. As seen in current practice, however, rickets usually presents because of stunting of stature and painful bones, and there is often only slight swelling over the epiphyseal regions.

Diagnosis of rickets. The results of investigation are similar to those of osteomalacia; the biochemical profile shows a low-normal or low serum calcium, a low inorganic phosphate and an elevated alkaline phosphatase. It must be remembered that the normal range for the latter estimation is much higher in the growing child than in the adult. The characteristic radiological features of rickets are broadening of the epiphyseal lines with cupping of the metaphysis. In extreme cases marked deformities of the shafts of the bone may be seen.

Treatment. This consists of giving vitamin D_3 to supplement the diet. A dose of 0·125 mg (5000 units) daily is usually sufficient in treatment. Assuming that the existing deficiency is corrected the best preventive is to take a diet which is adequate in calcium and vitamin D content (around 10 μg (400 units)/day).

Various other types of rickets are described but these are very much rarer than the nutritional rickets. These can be conveniently considered as:

1. Renal rickets. This is the condition of severe renal osteodystrophy in childhood and is discussed under that heading.
2. Vitamin D resistant rickets. This is characterised by a familial disorder in which there is short stature associated with evidence of clinical rickets and a low plasma inorganic phosphate level. It has been suggested in this disorder that the primary defect is either an inability to absorb calcium or an excessive loss of phosphate in the urine. The condition requires phosphate together with an active metabolite of Vitamin D for its treatment.
3. Rickets associated with primary renal tubular disorders such as the Fanconi syndrome and renal tubular acidosis.
4. Hypophosphatasia. This is a condition in which the clinical features of mild rickets are associated with lack of alkaline phosphatase in bone and plasma inherited as an autosomal recessive abnormality.

Renal osteodystrophy

It has been recognised for some time that bone problems may develop as a rare accompaniment to chronic renal failure. Such cases were considered rather as academic curiosities until the advent of large scale chronic renal dialysis programmes which enabled the maintenance of life in patients who would previously have died from renal failure. In such patients there is an increasing incidence of renal osteodystrophy although this does seem to vary from centre to centre. This variation has been postulated by some authors to reflect the vitamin D status of the individuals before they developed renal disease.

Clinically these patients present with bone pain and, if in the childhood age group, they present with the features of rickets, this being the condition of renal rickets.

Biochemically the changes are those expected in osteomalacia. There is a low serum calcium which is caused by failure of absorption of calcium from the gut and is often aggravated by a low level of plasma proteins. With the recent knowledge that the kidney plays an important role in producing an active form of vitamin D it is reasonable to postulate that in these patients there may be a defective formation of 1,25-dihydroxy vitamin D with resultant difficulties in absorption of calcium. The changes in serum inorganic phosphate are often difficult to interpret because there are two opposing forces. The renal failure tends to increase the serum inorganic phosphate level and secondary hyperparathyroidism, caused by the low serum calcium, tends to lower the serum inorganic phosphate by causing a phosphaturia. The results found in practice are, therefore, variable. There is however an elevated level of alkaline phosphatase because of the secondary hyperparathyroidism.

Radiologically there is a mixture of osteoporosis, osteomalacia because of the lack of vitamin D, and hyperparathyroidism because of the secondary parathyroid overactivity.

A similar conflicting picture is obtained on histological examination of a bone biopsy in which the changes of all three types of bone disease are seen.

Renal osteodystrophy therefore is a very complex bone problem which is usually recognised in the context of the renal lesion.

Treatment. It was recognised many years ago that children with renal rickets were very resistant to vitamin D. They required much larger doses than did children with nutritional rickets and this is now explicable on the basis of the failure of the kidney to synthesise active metabolites of vitamin D. 1–25 dihydroxyvitamin D or 1α hydroxyvitamin D in small doses are now used in preference to the previously employed large doses of vitamin D itself. Phosphate levels and the liability to metastatic calcification are controlled by giving oral phosphate binding agents such as aluminium hydroxide.

In the occasional patient, the secondary hyperparathyroidism may proceed to tertiary hyperparathyroidism and in such patients consideration may require to be given to the possibility of removal of a parathyroid adenoma. This condition will usually be suspected where the serum calcium is at upper normal or elevated levels in a patient with well established renal disease. This is a difficult therapeutic decision.

Paget's disease

Paget's disease of bone is a very common condition in older people. In this condition there is gross disorganisation of bone structure. The regular system of lamellar deposition of hydroxyapatite crystals is broken down and there is very active bone formation and bone destruction both proceeding at the same time. The condition was first described by Sir James Paget and initially only gross cases were recognised with softening and bending of the bones, broadening of the head and very frequently increasing deafness. This latter symptom is sometimes due to pressure on the auditory nerves due to thickening in the skull.

Apart from this very obvious clinical presentation the diagnosis of Paget's disease is very frequently made as an incidental finding in X-rays of the spine or pelvic bones done for some other purpose such as an I.V.P. or a barium meal. Sometimes it is made following the finding of an isolated elevated serum alkaline phosphatase. Yet other patients may present because of pain in a bone often associated with swelling, localised to the region of pain, with a noticeable increase in skin temperature over the affected bone. Bones affected by Paget's disease are liable to pathological fracture.

The diagnosis of Paget's disease is made on the finding of the typical radiological picture of marked coarsening and sclerosis of the affected bones. The trabeculae are characteristically disorganised. The changes may affect the whole skeleton or may affect only one isolated bone. Involvement of one bone is of course unusual in the other metabolic bone diseases where usually the process is a diffuse one. A radioisotope scan of bone is the most sensitive method for detecting areas of Paget's disease.

The biochemical findings in Paget's disease are a normal serum calcium, although this on occasion may be slightly raised, a normal serum inorganic phosphate and a very marked elevation in the serum alkaline phosphatase. The urinary hydroxyproline values are elevated.

Histologically the bone shows gross disorganisation of structure but histology is not required to make the diagnosis.

Treatment. The treatment of Paget's disease of bone has been improved by the advent of calcitonin. Since calcitonin works by preventing breakdown of bone it is an ideal treatment for Paget's disease where there is an overactive breakdown and reformation of bone. The administration of calcitonin allows restoration of virtually normal bony structure with the relief of bone pain. Both porcine and salmon calcitonin are available as synthetic preparations for parenteral administration. Calcitonin requires to be given by intramuscular injection since it is a protein hormone and in a few patients there is an anaphylactoid reaction to it.

It is not clear which patients with Paget's disease should be treated with calcitonin. There is general agreement that those patients with bone pain or any other acute bone problem should receive treatment but it does not seem logical to treat those patients in whom the diagnosis is made as an incidental finding and who are asymptomatic. Other lines of therapy involve the use of diphosphonates, fluoride and mithramycin.

One complication of Paget's disease is that of sarcomatous change. Malignant change, however, must be very rare when one takes into account the high incidence of Paget's disease in the elderly population.

Osteopetrosis

Osteopetrosis is the opposite condition from osteoporosis. In osteopetrosis there is increased bone density. It, as already mentioned, occurs with the chronic ingestion of fluoride in toxic doses. There is, however, a number of other conditions which occur as uncommon sporadic diseases and in which there is increased density of the bones. It might seem reasonable to think that some of these conditions may be due to increased levels of calcitonin with resultant inhibition of the normal bone breakdown. However, there has been no evidence of increased levels of serum calcitonin in most patients with osteopetrosis. The only exception was a case report of a woman with excessive levels of calcitonin due to a medullary carcinoma of the thyroid who gave birth to children affected by osteopetrosis.

There is no specific treatment that is known to influence osteopetrosis.

Osteogenesis imperfecta (fragilitas ossium)

This is a condition in which there is a defect in the formation of bone matrix, that is, a defect in collagen formation and not a primary disorder of calcification. This disorder occurs in a variety of forms, one of which may be very severe and may affect the child in utero so that the infant is born with multiple fractures. In other instances the disease is much more benign and this degree of clinical disorder is compatible with survival until adult life. Apart from marked thinning of the bones seen on X-ray, the classical feature which should raise suspicion of this disorder is the presence of blue sclerae. The blueness of the sclerae is due to the thinness of collagen in the scleral layers allowing the black pigment of the choroidal layer to show through as a modified blue colour. It should be noted, however, that not all patients with osteogenesis imperfecta have blue sclerae. In fact many patients who are severely affected do not show any alteration in the eyes.

The main clinical problem in these patients is pathological fractures. There is no specific therapy which influences the underlying bone disorder itself.

Achondroplasia

In this condition there is defective formation of bone derived from cartilage as opposed to membranous bone. In these patients therefore the bones of the head, spine and trunk are normally formed whereas the limb bones are abnormal and are very short. The disorder is an inherited one but assuming the patient so affected survives through infancy there is a reasonably normal life span. Most patients with this disorder are strong and apart from their short stature and abnormally short length of limbs compared to trunk show no obvious defects. Many are indeed employed as circus dwarfs. There is no treatment which will influence the stature of these patients.

FURTHER READING

Symposium 1974 Parathyroid hormone, calcitonin and vitamin D. American Journal of Medicine 56: 743, 57: 1

Avioli L V, Raisz L G 1980 Metabolic bone disease. Clinics in Endocrinology and Metabolism 9: 1

Buckle R 1974 Disorders of the parathyroid glands. Clinics in Endocrinology and Metabolism 3: 2

Nordin B E C 1973 Osteoporosis. Clinics in Endocrinology and Metabolism 2: 2

Nordin B E C 1973 Metabolic Bone and Stone Disease. Churchill Livingstone, Edinburgh

9

Obesity; hirsutism; disorders of the breast

It is proposed in this chapter to review certain diseases which present commonly to an endocrine clinic but which are not attributable to dysfunction of a particular endocrine organ.

OBESITY

This is one of the most common referrals to the endocrinologist. It is difficult to give an absolute definition of obesity. Common methods of definition have been based on the comparison of the patient's weight with an 'ideal' body weight, often an excess of 20 per cent over the 'ideal' weight being taken as representing obesity: an alternative method attempts to measure the proportion of fat by estimating the skin fold thickness over areas such as over the triceps muscle or over the back as an index of obesity. In the obese patient referred to an endocrine clinic difficulties in defining obesity do not arise as the patients are grossly overweight even by the most casual inspection. The majority of patients with obesity are female.

Obesity is an important condition since it is associated with a considerable increase in the rate of morbidity and mortality from such conditions as diabetes mellitus, gall bladder disease, hypertension and atherosclerosis. The reason for referral to the endocrinologist is that the patient, like her doctor, is hopeful of finding some glandular cause to explain excessive weight gain, which is most often clearly due to excessive calorie intake and lack of exercise. It must be admitted that in a few patients an endocrine cause will be found. Such a cause is to be expected since the hypothalamus is one of the important centres for integrating appetite and thirst, and the adrenal and the thyroid glands obviously play a major role in the metabolic processes. It must be emphasised, however, that in the vast majority of overweight patients there is no demonstrable endocrine dysfunction to which the obesity can be attributed. Even in patients with an endocrine problem such as hypothyroidism or Cushing's syndrome although the weight increases, the degree of weight gain is not gross. Usually clinical examination alone will suffice to exclude adrenal or thyroid disease and aided by the appropriate biochemical and radiological investigations endocrine diseases can be firmly excluded. While it is important not to miss remediable endocrine disease one must not keep on repeatedly investigating the obese patient in the vain hope of turning up some endocrine condition.

It is important that an accurate dietary history is taken. Most patients initially claim to eat very little or to take one meal a day. Closer questioning reveals that this 'diet' in fact adds up to a large number of calories, often in the form of carbohydrate, inappropriate to the degree of energy expenditure. Some patients will admit to eating in binges and others to constant nibbling of snacks rather than eating regular large meals. One must be aware of the contribution of soft drinks and alcohol to the total calorie intake.

The clinical examination of the obese patient usually reveals a gross generalised pattern of obesity. The patient, if middle-aged, may well be hypertensive. Often in the young there is confusion with Cushing's syndrome. If weight gain has been recent and rapid, especially round about puberty, some fine striae, red in colour, may be found round the buttocks and the breasts. These striae look quite unlike the broad striae of Cushing's syndrome. Furthermore the skin of the obese patient is not atrophic. It has been noted elsewhere that children obese because of overnutrition are tall for their chronological age whereas the patient with glucocorticoid excess is stunted.

Treatment

Theoretically weight loss could be achieved by reducing calorie intake, altering the digestive process, preventing absorption of nutrients or altering the metabolism. Of these options the one most readily available is to control the calorie intake. Once appropriate investigations have been performed it is essential to have the patient's co-operation in following a reduction dietary regime usually of around 800 to 1000 calories. The dietician has an important role in the management of the obese patient and should go over the prescribed diet in detail. Usually if the patient co-operates in dieting, weight loss takes place. Many patients have an unrealistic expectation of the rate of weight loss. It must be made clear to them that a loss of 0·5–1Kg/week is very satisfactory provided that this is regularly achieved. In a few patients the obesity is apparently intractable. It is then useful to admit them for a short time to hospital to cause more rapid initial weight loss by very strict dieting. Their response to such a regime encourages them and demonstrates that it is indeed possible to lose weight by dieting. The long term benefits of very prolonged in-patient dieting are disappointing as most patients are likely to put on weight again on leaving hospital. In some refractory patients regimes of complete starvation have been used but these are associated with significant morbidity and occasional mortality.

Once an appropriate degree of weight loss has been obtained it is vital to try to get the patient to adhere to a suitable long term diet. The more the diet can be made to approximate to the patient's normal type of food the better and more likely is she to adhere to it.

The use of appetite suppressants is controversial. The general experience is that although they might be useful in helping to obtain initial weight loss in patients apparently resistant to dieting, they are not a good long term treatment. Often their use results in the patient becoming psychologically dependent on her pills. Many even come to regard the taking of appetite suppressant pills as an adequate substitute for following an appropriate diet!

In a small number of very intractable obese patients more drastic manoeuvres such as splinting the teeth together or various types of bowel short circuiting operations have been undertaken. These latter operative procedures result in iatrogenic steatorrhoea which allows the patients to eat relatively freely but exposes them to the risk of vitamin deficiency because of malabsorption. The long term value of this treatment is not clear.

HIRSUTISM

The presence of excessive hair in the female is another common cause of referral to an endocrine clinic. What is often not realised is that there is a very wide variation in the amount of hair normally present in the female. Racial differences in amounts of hair may be noted. Some Asiatic races have noticeably less hair than the Europeans, especially those from southern Europe. Many hirsute females will admit to other female members of the family also being affected.

In dealing with a hirsute patient the first essential is to establish whether or not the patient's complaint of excessive hair is really justified. It should be emphasised that it is not abnormal for a female to have some coarse hairs round the nipples or to have a few coarse hairs in the midline of the chest. It is also common for the so-called male distribution of pubic hair to be seen in the female, that is the pubic hair extending upwards in the midline towards the umbilicus and not terminating in a horizontal upper border. Age is another important factor in that it is common for women after the menopause to develop additional facial hair often on the chin or on the upper lip. All these factors, therefore, should be taken into account before concluding that the amount of hair present is abnormal. What is often found is that the patient's reaction to her 'normal' amount of hair is abnormal. Sometimes this may amount to a frankly obsessional state.

Assuming, however, that the doctor agrees with the patient that the distribution or amount of hair present is abnormal, the next thing is to try and make an assessment of the likely source of stimulus to hair growth. Details of the menstrual cycle should be obtained since, if regular menstruation is occurring, a marked excess of androgen production is unlikely. The patient should have a general examination with particular attention to muscle build since good muscular development with little subcutaneous fat suggests androgen excess especially if combined with loss of the scalp hair and frontal baldness of male type. Examination of the external genitalia should be made for any sign of clitoral enlargement. In all significantly hirsute patients a gynaecological assessment should be obtained. Depending on the clinical findings this may range from simple pelvic examination to more complex procedures to demonstrate the ovaries such as laparoscopy, gynaecography and laparotomy.

An assessment of androgen production should be undertaken: the particular tests used will depend on the facilities available. Appropriate tests would include estimation of the urinary 17-oxosteroids (17-ketosteroids) which gives a crude index of the total androgen excretion or preferably measurement of the plasma testosterone. If elevated levels are found, these estimations may be combined with suppression tests with either dexamethasone or oestrogens to suppress the adrenal and ovarian function. While it might be thought that dexamethasone would suppress only the adrenals it has been shown that it can also suppress the ovarian production of androgenic hormones. This effect may be explained by the common origin of both the adrenal and the ovary from the mesonephric ridge.

In addition to estimation of the plasma testosterone, estimation of the sex hormone binding globulin should ideally be performed. It is theoretically possible to have a low testosterone due to a pathologically low sex hormone binding globulin which results in an elevated free testosterone level.

Once these various tests have been performed, one should be in a position to diagnose or exclude significant endocrine disease such as:

1. *Ovarian disease*. Most commonly hirsutism of ovarian origin is due to the polycystic ovarian syndrome which should be treated in the manner outlined in the chapter on the ovary. It may rarely be due to ovarian tumours which should be removed. Some ovarian tumours such as the hilus cell tumour are so small that to exclude them

completely one may need to bisect the ovary at operation.

2. *Adrenal disease* in the form of Cushing's syndrome with mixed glucocorticoid and androgen excess or rarely due to virilising adrenal tumours should be treated as outlined in the chapter on the adrenal. Patients who have one of the enzymatic defects of the adrenal gland should be on glucocorticoid suppressive therapy.

3. *Iatrogenic disease* due to the administration of androgenic drugs.

Once these conditions are excluded one is left with the majority of patients who do not fall into any of these categories and who are, therefore, examples of idiopathic hirsutism. In many of these patients there is some evidence of slight androgen excess and it is possible in these patients that there are minor defects of cortisol synthesis with minor over-production of androgens as a result of compensatory adjustment by the adrenal. An alternative explanation, for which there is no good evidence, is that the hair follicles of the hirsute patient respond excessively to physiological amounts of androgen.

The great problem in the management of hirsutism is what to do with this group of patients with idiopathic hirsutism. Treatment may be considered in the following categories.

1. Local cosmetic treatment. This can be with various types of hair removing creams, waxes, electrolysis, shaving or bleaching. The choice of method depends on the area affected, it being well recognised that on the face prolonged use of waxes or hair removing creams results in severe irritation. Electrolysis is effective where there are comparatively few coarse hairs to be removed but is not very effective when the area of abnormal hair is very large. Where there is a large amount of hair to be removed there is no doubt that shaving is probably the simplest method although many women dislike the idea of using any form of razor.

2. Attempts to suppress abnormal androgen production where this can be demonstrated and where there is no evidence of an ovarian or adrenal tumour. In those patients who respond to oestrogen, it is reasonable to attempt long term suppression of the excess androgen by one of the oestrogen-containing oral contraceptive drugs. The alternative treatment by dexamethasone to suppress the adrenal and/or the ovary, although attractive biochemically, has major drawbacks: it is difficult to justify the prolonged use of a potent glucocorticoid preparation with all its attendant side-effects in the treatment of a cosmetic problem. Anti-androgen drugs such as cyproterone acetate which is said to block the uptake of testosterone by the hair follicle is now in clinical use but its exact value in the treatment of hirsutism remains to be defined.

DISORDERS OF THE BREAST

Galactorrhoea has already been discussed in the chapter on the hypothalamus and pituitary but other breast disorders are seen by the endocrinologist. Of these the most common is gynaecomastia. Studies have shown that a minor degree of breast enlargement in the male is a not uncommon condition when specific clinical and histological examination is made, but clinically significant gynaecomastia is comparatively uncommon (Table 8.1).

Table 8.1 Causes of gynaecomastia

a) Physiological—puberty
b) Liver disease
c) Drugs such as spironolactone, cimetidine and oestrogen
d) Refeeding gynaecomastia
e) Endocrine disease
    1) Thyrotoxicosis
    2) Pituitary tumours producing prolactin
    3) Feminising tumour of adrenal or testis
    4) Testicular tumour producing HCG
f) Chromosomal—Klinefelter's syndrome

The commonest type is 'pubertal' gynaecomastia, so-called from its appearance around the time of puberty. Usually it is of mild degree and settles down without therapy but sometimes it persists and can be a major source of embarrassment in the adolescent boy. Gynaecomastia in the absence of galactorrhoea seems to be associated with excess oestrogen formation probably due to the interconversion of androgen to oestrogen rather than due to excessive prolactin. In these cases of gynaecomastia without galactorrhoea it is noticeable that the nipple is not developed as it is when prolactin is present in excess.

The other common cause of gynaecomastia in the male is liver disease: it is postulated that this condition is due to the failure of the liver to detoxicate circulating oestrogens.

Gynaecomastia is also seen in other general medical conditions such as in patients on regular renal dialysis. This latter condition is of interest: it is thought to be similar in origin to the so-called re-feeding gynaecomastia that was described in prisoners of war who developed gynaecomastia as a sudden phenomenon when their nutritional status was improved as a result of an increased protein and calorie intake. It is probably in consequence of increased gonadotrophin production in these patients.

The therapeutic administration of oestrogen in prostatic carcinoma or self therapy in homosexual patients produces breast enlargement. Similarly, in rare instances gynaecomastia may be due to oestrogen-producing tumours of the adrenal or testes. Apart from the administration of female sex hormones, other drugs, notably spironolactone and drugs implicated in the causation of galactorrhoea, may cause gynaecomastia.

Endocrine disease is not a common cause of gynaecomastia. Perhaps the most common endocrine cause is thyrotoxicosis. Other much less common causes are the oestrogen producing tumours already mentioned and chorioephithelioma of testis which produces HCG. In Klinefelter's syndrome the gynaecomastia is also thought to be due to the increased gonadotrophin production.

In noting breast enlargement in the male it should be remembered that breast carcinoma can be found in male patients especially in those with an abnormal karyotype such as 47 XXY. In this instance the gynaecomastia would be unilateral.

The treatment of gynaecomastia is to remove the underlying cause and deal with any endocrine disease present. Otherwise the treatment is plastic surgery to remove the excessive breast tissue.

The antigonadotrophic agent, danazol, has been claimed to be successful in the treatment of pubertal gynaecomastia but it must be remembered that most cases settle spontaneously.

Other breast disorders

In addition to the relatively common conditions such as galactorrhoea or gynaecomastia the endocrinologist is asked to see other patients with breast conditions. These are often patients who have a marked discrepancy in the development of each breast, some indeed with development completely absent on one side. There is no evidence that this anomaly is due to any endocrine disease. The only treatment for it is plastic surgery to adjust the discrepancy by doing either an augmentation mammoplasty on the smaller side or a reduction mammoplasty on the larger.

Another group of patients seen are apparently normal women who are dissatisfied with the size of their breasts. There is no evidence that giving such patients female sex hormones makes any difference to the breast size. Almost certainly they have normal circulating oestrogen levels and this can be easily confirmed biochemically. Their existing breast size is that determined by the responsiveness of the breast tissue to these oestrogens and it is not augmented by exogenous oestrogen administration. If they are particularly concerned about their condition they should be referred for treatment by plastic surgery as it is fairly simple to perform an augmentation mammoplasty.

FURTHER READING

Abe K 1980 Endocrinology and cancer. Clinics in Endocrinology and Metabolism 9: 2
Rees L H, Ratcliffe J G 1974 Ectopic hormone production by non-endocrine tumours. Clinical Endocrinology 3: 263

10

Endocrine syndromes caused by non-endocrine tumours

INTRODUCTION

Although the clinical association of adrenocortical hyperplasia with bronchial carcinoma was recognised almost 50 years ago it is only recently that there has been a major interest in the endocrine effects of non-endocrine tumours. One of the main reasons for this interest is the increasing availability of more sophisticated laboratory techniques which allow assay not only of the end organ hormones produced from endocrine glands and non-endocrine tumours but of stimulatory hormones such as ACTH, TSH etc. released by these tumours. There is no doubt that when a deliberate search for endocrine abnormalities is made amongst patients suffering from carcinomata these are found in a large number. It is, however, also true that in most cases the clinical manifestations of these biochemical abnormalities are not florid and only a few patients will be recognised during life as having clinical disease in relation to the endocrine system. Indeed with current assay techniques used to study not only the patient's blood but also tumour tissue resected at operation or removed at post mortem, it is recognised that more than one endocrine abnormality may be found associated with many tumours and tumours secreting four or more different hormones have been described.

The mechanism of production of these biochemical abnormalities is of great interest not merely in the field of endocrinology but in attempting to expand our understanding of the control of cell function. Various possibilities exist:

1. That the ectopic hormone production is a manifestation of derepression of the cell control mechanisms during the de-differentiation which occurs as part of the malignant process. Thus according to this theory every cell has the potentiality to secrete all peptide hormones since every cell has the same content of DNA. It is thought that the fact that the one cell does not produce a variety of hormones in the normal subject is because only one part of the DNA molecule is allowed to express itself and thereby stimulate peptide

production in any particular organ. During dedifferentiation it is therefore possible that more DNA might be freed from the repressing influences and thus more hormones be able to be produced. These hormones would theoretically be of a normal structure. This is the most favoured theory currently.

2. It might be argued that during tumour formation the cell has acquired a new ability to secrete peptide hormones rather than the unmasking of a potentiality as described in 1 above. It is, however, possible as an extension of this argument that the ectopic peptide hormones produced in tumour tissue are not of entirely normal structure and thus although they may exert biochemical effects, they are able to be identified on radioimmunoassay techniques as being immunologically unlike the normal hormone.

3. It is possible that the tumours do not actually produce the hormones at all but may merely have the ability to collect normal hormone secretions from the blood flowing through them. An argument against this, however, is that if one assays the arterial and venous blood supplying a tumour-bearing organ one is usually able to note a difference in concentration between the two samples, the venous sample being of higher hormone concentration than the arterial sample thus suggesting that the tumour is releasing the hormone to the blood. Furthermore *in vitro* tissue culture studies have shown tumours can actually form the hormones and secrete them into the medium.

Clinical syndromes produced by ectopic hormone formation

1. *Ectopic ACTH syndrome.* This is by far the most widely recognised ectopic hormone syndrome in man and the majority of cases are due to a bronchial carcinoma particularly of oat cell variety. Ectopic ACTH production has, however, been described in relation to tumours of other organs such as thymus, pancreas and medullary carcinoma of the thyroid. In the ectopic ACTH syndrome there is a clinical conflict between one disease process, bronchial carcinoma causing wasting, and the ectopic ACTH syndrome causing Cushing's syndrome with associated weight gain. Because of this modification of the clinical picture of spontaneous Cushing's syndrome, i.e. that due to adrenal or pituitary disease, the clinical findings in the ectopic ACTH syndrome are not usually so florid. The diagnosis is therefore usually made on the basis of the biochemical findings although the occasional patient may show sufficient signs such as facial plethora, pigmentation and peripheral oedema to draw clinical attention to the possibility of the disease. The possibility of the ectopic ACTH syndrome should be particularly kept in mind when dealing with

clinical or biochemical Cushing's syndrome in middle aged males in view of the high incidence of bronchial carcinoma in this group.

The diagnosis is, however, often made in the context of first diagnosing a patient as having a bronchial carcinoma and then recognising on routine biochemical testing that a marked hypokalaemic alkalosis exists. From this starting point plasma cortisol estimations are performed and these will be found to be extremely high. When the endocrine investigations are taken further it will be shown that the blood ACTH levels are also very high, indeed much higher than that found in Cushing's syndrome caused by hypothalamic/pituitary disease. The appropriate treatment is to treat the primary tumour by surgery or radiotherapy where this is feasible. Where this is not possible treatment with opDDD, metyrapone or aminoglutethamide may induce temporary benefit.

2. *Inappropriate ADH secretion* (Schwartz-Bartter syndrome). This is another abnormality which is often recognised in the context of bronchial carcinoma although it can be found in the presence of non-malignant disease of the chest including certain pneumonias. The patient is usually unwell because of the primary illness and is typically confused. On electrolyte screening he is found to have a marked dilutional pattern of the plasma electrolytes with a low sodium, potassium, chloride and urea. When the plasma osmolality is measured it will be found to be below normal, although the urine is hypertonic. This syndrome is treated by curing the primary disease where this is possible. If this is not feasible these patients are best managed by water deprivation. It is of no benefit to give salt to correct the hyponatraemia as this merely increases the fluid retention. Recently lithium has been described as having a diuretic effect on water excretion by the renal tubules and this might be one possible means of treatment.

3. *Hypercalcaemic syndromes*. Various tumours are associated with hypercalcaemia. By far the commonest cause of hypercalcaemia in association with non-endocrine tumours is the presence of metastatic bone disease. This can sometimes be difficult to diagnose and may require repeated bone scanning or bone biopsy to prove because on some occasions radiological skeletal survey may not be diagnostic. If, however, one can exclude those cases who have metastatic bone disease, there remains a number of patients with hypercalcaemia associated with non-endocrine tumours. In some of these it appears that the tumour is producing a parathormone-like hormone (pseudohyperparathyroidism) and in others it appears that it is producing a vitamin D-like steroid. The end point of both of these states is of course to cause hypercalcaemia and the importance of

recognising that this is present is that often the patient's symptoms of hypercalcaemia which are nausea, vomiting, anorexia, constipation and mental impairment may be attributed to metastatic tumour whereas they are in fact caused by an endocrine effect which may be amenable to therapy. Hypercalcaemia, when it is at emergency levels, can be reduced by infusing phosphate or sulphate but probably the most hopeful long term therapy in these patients is to use calcitonin or steroid therapy.

4. *Thyrotoxicosis* due to ectopic production of TSH-like hormones has been described as an uncommon entity especially in association with chorioepithelioma. This finding is explicable on the basis that the normal placenta produces a TSH-like hormone. Recent work has suggested that the thyroid stimulating substance may simply be human chorionic gonadotrophin (HCG) itself. This hormone has a weak thyroid stimulating effect but is present in chorioepithelioma in such quantitites that this effect can be clinically significant. In such patients biochemical and occasional clinical thyrotoxicosis may be found. Treatment is to remove the primary tumour where this is feasible or to treat by cytotoxic drugs.

5. *Hypoglycaemia*. This has been recognised in association with tumours of various organs apart from diseases of the pancreas. The best known of these are large retroperitoneal soft tissue tumours but it has also been described in cases of hepatoma. The mechanism of production of the hypoglycaemia by these tumours is not clear. It has been suggested that this may be simply due to the tumour metabolising large amounts of glucose but it is also possible that these tumours may be producing an insulin-like material and indeed such a substance is able to be measured by bioassay procedures from certain tumours. The hypoglycaemic symptoms respond to resection of the tumour where this is feasible.

6. *Polycythaemia*. Although not usually considered an endocrine disease, polycythaemia has been recognised for some years to be associated with malignant tumours and benign conditions of the kidney. Polycythaemia has also been associated with a rare brain tumour, cerebellar haemangioblastoma.

The kidney normally manufactures a hormone, erythropoietin, which passes to the bone marrow and stimulates it to produce red cells. In polycythaemia it is attractive to argue that this stimulus may be excessive and this explains the polycythaemia of renal tumours. In contrast to the more common primary polycythaemia the polycythaemia secondary to a renal lesion typically shows no associated rise in white cell or platelet count. The polycythaemia in such cases can be cured by nephrectomy.

7. *Other ectopic hormones*. In addition to the above well recognised conditions newer assays have revealed that other hormones are commonly produced in non-endocrine tumours. Examples of such hormones are calcitonin and growth hormone. In particular calcitonin has been found to be commonly associated with metastatic carcinoma of breast. The clinical role of these in patients with carcinoma remains to be defined.

FURTHER READING

Abe K 1980 Endocrinology and cancer. Clinics in Endocrinology and Metabolism 9: 2

Rees L H, Ratcliffe J G 1974 Ectopic hormone production by non-endocrine tumours. Clinical Endocrinology 3: 263

11

Clinical syndromes caused by abnormal secretion of gastrointestinal hormones

INTRODUCTION

Classical descriptions of gastrointestinal physiology abound with names of substances such as gastrin, enterogastrone, cholecystokinin, secretin and pancreozymin, which are all names given to extracts of various portions of the gastrointestinal mucosa which exert modulating effects on other aspects of gastrointestinal function.

In some cases the experimental effects are produced by no specific identifiable chemical substance but for others, such as gastrin, we have a much clearer idea of the identity of the substance under consideration. Problems which have presented themselves in trying to define roles for gastrointestinal hormones have been (a) the biochemical variability of the hormone itself even when there is reasonable chemical identification such as in the case of gastrin. This hormone appears to occur in a variety of forms of different molecular size making it difficult to say which particular molecular species is the physiologically important one. (b) In many cases the hormones exert their effects on the gastrointestinal tract not by a systemic route but by a local effect on an adjacent area of the gut and are, therefore, not readily available for isolation and assay.

It is, however, clear that the gastrointestinal tract is a major endocrine organ which has been comparatively neglected until recently. This deficiency is now being repaired with the description of a variety of clinical endocrine conditions associated with excess production of gastrointestinal hormones.

Where do these hormones come from? The weight of the current evidence is that the hormone-producing cells of the gastrointestinal tract, which of course includes the pancreas with its well known local areas of endocrine cells—the islets of Langerhans—come from the primitive neural crest. These cells have common cytochemical properties and are described as APUD cells (amine precursor uptake and decarboxylation). Cells of this type occur at many sites throughout the length of the gastrointestinal tract and therefore the gut constitutes a diffuse endocrine organ rather than a localised mass of endocrine tissue like the thryoid. This contributes to the problems of isolating the gut hormones in pure form.

The clinical syndromes

There are at present 5 main syndromes recognised to be associated with excess production of gastrointestinal hormones.

1. Zollinger-Ellison syndrome (ZE syndrome), gastrinoma
2. Glucagonoma
3. Insulinoma
4. Pancreatic cholera (watery diarrhoea, hypokalaemia, achlorhydria syndrome, WDHA syndrome or Verner-Morrison syndrome)
5. Carcinoid syndrome

1. *Zollinger-Ellison syndrome (gastrinoma)*

This is the condition produced by an adenoma of the pancreatic islet tissue which is releasing a large amount of gastrin. There is controversy about which pancreatic islet cell gives rise to a gastrinoma as gastrin is not produced by the normal pancreas. This hormone is released in the physiological state from the antral tissue of the stomach and acts to stimulate the production of pepsin and hydrochloric acid from the fundal area of the stomach. Its release, under physiological conditions, seems to be under both local and neural control. The local control is effected by alteration of pH in the gastric contents coming into contact with the antral mucosa. Where these contents are of high acidity gastrin secretion is diminished: where the pH rises gastrin secretion is stimulated. However, gastrin secretion also can be activated by the sight, taste or smell of food and this influence seems to be mediated by the vagus nerve.

In the pathological condition of a gastrin-secreting tumour (gastrinoma) there is an autonomous over-production of gastrin and, therefore, one of the major clinical manifestations which can be anticipated from physiological considerations is the production of severe intractable peptic ulceration of the stomach, duodenum and jejunum with often multiple ulcers being present. Characteristically when these ulcers are not recognised as being due to underlying gastrin hypersecretion, they recur very shortly after gastric surgery. Apart from ulceration the other change of note in the stomach is hypertrophy of the rugae of the gastric fundus because of the trophic effect of gastrin on the mucosa.

The other major symptom associated with a gastrinoma is diarrhoea which can at times result in massive fluid loss from the gut. The actual mechanism of production of the diarrhoea is not clear but it is probably related to the profound pH changes in the bowel contents as the result of the hypersecretion of acid in the stomach. Steatorrhoea is also characteristically found. This has been attributed to inhibition of pancreatic lipase activity due to the prevailing low intestinal pH as a result of gastric hyperacidity.

Diagnosis depends on the demonstration of a high basal acid secretion and on the demonstration of multiple peptic ulceration and gross hypertrophy of the rugae of the stomach, found either on upper gastrointestinal radiology or on endoscopy. The diagnosis is confirmed by estimation of the serum gastrin in the fasting state. Normal ranges for serum gastrin are <100ng/l, often with values of 10 times this in patients with gastrinoma.

In borderline cases various stimulatory tests of gastrin secretion using secretin or calcium infusion have been used but their place in the diagnosis of gastrinoma is controversial.

It should be noted that an elevated gastrin level by itself does not necessarily indicate a gastrinoma as raised levels have been found in association with atrophic gastritis, pernicious anaemia, renal failure, gastric ulcer and during the use of drugs such as anticholinergics and H_2-receptor antagonists which block acid secretion.

In some cases, the tumour can be localised by coeliac axis angiography but often a gastrinoma is quite small and may not be shown by radiological techniques.

Treatment consists of resection of the pancreatic adenoma if possible although it must be borne in mind that approximately two-thirds of these tumours are malignant and result in metastatic disease. The alternative surgical treatment is total gastrectomy. More recently the condition has been shown to be amenable to treatment with cimetidine, an H_2-receptor antagonist, and thus the place of total gastrectomy has diminished.

2. *Glucagonoma*

As its name suggests this is a tumour of the alpha cells of the islets of Langerhans producing excess glucagon. This tumour does not produce a distinct endocrine syndrome but its diagnosis may be suspected from the presence of mild diabetes mellitus and skin lesions, the typical one being a necrotic lesion of skin, necrolytic migratory erythema. The diagnosis is confirmed by the demonstration of high levels of circulating glucagon.

In addition to cases of glucagonoma, cases are described which have excess production of glucagon from a diffuse hyperplasia of the islet cells.

As in a gastrinoma many of these glucagon-secreting tumours are malignant and require appropriate surgical removal.

3. *Insulinoma*

This has been already dealt with in the chapter on disturbances of carbohydrate metabolism.

4. *Pancreatic cholera*

This name has been given to a clinical syndrome of severe watery diarrhoea which is associated with severe hypokalaemia and which may indeed be severe enough to lead to renal failure. This was the mechanism of death in the original two cases diagnosed at post mortem. In this respect the severe watery diarrhoea is similar to that found in the Zollinger-Ellison syndrome but in contrast to that syndrome instead of being associated with an excessive production of acid from the stomach there is, in pancreatic cholera, severe hypochlorhydria and even achlorhydria in some patients. Other features of the condition are flushing of the skin and hypercalcaemia. The causation of this latter feature is not known.

The mechanism of production of the severe diarrhoea is also not clear. Various gastrointestinal hormones have been suggested as the cause. The most favoured at present is vasoactive intestinal peptide (VIP), but others may be associated with a similar clinical syndrome. The diagnosis is, therefore, made on the basis of the clinical picture and confirmed by measurement of the serum VIP levels. Since often it is associated with a pancreatic adenoma larger than that found in the Zollinger-Ellison syndrome the diagnosis may be confirmed by coeliac axis arteriography. Treatment is surgical removal of the pancreatic tumour following correction of the electrolyte imbalance. As with other pancreatic adenomata malignant change can occur.

5. *Carcinoid syndrome*

This is a well recognised although rare condition in which tumours at many points in the gastrointestinal tract, particularly in the small bowel, are associated with endocrine effects. The term carcinoid was given to describe the contrast between the apparently malignant nature of the tumour on pathological examination and the comparatively low rate of growth when followed clinically. Characteristically, the clinical features are of flushing, diarrhoea, abdominal pain and the presence of cardiac lesions on the right side of the heart. In most cases there are large hepatic metastases present before such symptoms are produced. This is because the vasoactive peptides require access to the systemic circulation to produce symptoms. In the absence of hepatic metastases such peptides from the primary bowel tumour are detoxicated in the liver. This also explains why bronchial carcinoids can produce endocrine symptoms without the presence of hepatic metastases.

At one time the flush was thought to be produced by 5-hydroxytryptamine (serotonin) but in fact the present evidence would favour the flushing being induced by other vasoactive peptides such as bradykinin and kallikrein. The flush can be reproduced by various manoeuvres including the ingestion of alcohol which may provide a diagnostic clue.

The diagnosis is made by estimation of the urinary 5-hydroxyindoleacetic acid (5HIAA) which is the breakdown product of 5-hydroxytryptamine. Some tumours may produce related chemical substances such as 5-hydroxytryptophan instead of 5HIAA. The treatment is surgical resection of the primary tumour and as much of the metastases as is feasible. Various pharmacological agents including streptozotocin and methysergide have been tried with partial effect.

Additional abnormalities associated with the excess production of gastrointestinal hormones

a) Somatostatinoma: a small number of patients have been described with a tumour of the pancreas producing somatostatin. As expected from its anti-insulin action these patients were mildly diabetic.

b) Other apparent hormones from the gastrointestinal tract not only concerned with secretory function such as pancreatic polypeptide but also with bowel motility such as motilin have been described. The place which these and some of the more established hormones play in the physiology of the gastrointestinal tract or in the causation of common gastrointestinal diseases such as peptic ulcer or diarrhoeal states remains to be established.

Multiple endocrine neoplasia associated with endocrine tumours of the gastrointestinal tract

These endocrine relationships are explicable on the basis of the common embryological origin of the tissues giving rise to these tumours. They are clinically grouped into three syndromes called multiple endocrine neoplasia type 1 (Wermer's syndrome), multiple endocrine neoplasia type 2 (Sipple's syndrome) and a subgroup of type 2 referred to as type 3.

In MEN type 1 there is the association of tumours of the pituitary, parathyroid, adrenal, thyroid, carcinoid tumours and pancreatic tumours producing excess gastrin.

In MEN type 2 there is the simultaneous or consecutive production of medullary carcinoma of thyroid, parathyroid hyperplasia which may be a reaction to this hypocalcaemic stimulus, and phaeochromocytomas.

MEN type 3 is where there is the association of medullary carcinoma of the thyroid, phaeochromocytoma, a marfanoid facies and multiple mucosal neuromas. The disorder appears to be inherited as an autosomal dominant gene. Thus it is of value to use measurements of serum calcitonin in apparently unaffected relatives of an affected patient to try to diagnose medullary carcinoma of the thyroid at an early and treatable stage.

In these syndromes the endocrine tumours can become manifest only over a period of time and these associations should be borne in mind when a patient presents with one aspect of the syndrome. The treatment of these multiple endocrinopathies depends on which clinical feature is most prominent at any given time and such patients require skilled endocrine management over many years.

FURTHER READING

Bonfils S 1974 Endocrine-secreting tumours of the G I tract. Clinics in Gastroenterology 3: 3

Buchanan K D 1979 Gastrointestinal hormones. Clinics in Endocrinology and Metabolism 8: 2

Appendix

Values of laboratory tests commonly used in endocrinology

Note: there will be slight variations from laboratory to laboratory.

Thyroid

Serum total thyroxine 60–150 nmol/l
Serum total triiodothyronine 1–3 nmol/l
Serum TSH 0–8 mU/l
TRH test—increment of serum TSH to between 5–25 mU/l

Adrenal

Plasma 'cortisol' 300–700 nmol/l (evening plasma 'cortisol' <400 nmol/l)
Synacthen test—increment of plasma 'cortisol' > 200 nmol/l with 30 minute value > 550 nmol/l
Urinary free 'cortisol' < 1000 nmol/24 h
Urinary 17 oxosteroids 20–70 μmol/24 h
Urinary 17-hydroxycorticosteroids 15–50 μmol/24 h
Urinary metadrenalines 1·6–4·7 μmol/24 h

Gonadal

Plasma oestradiol

1. male 15–308 pmol/l
2. female (follicular phase) 200–1500 pmol/l
3. female (luteal phase) 450–800 pmol/l

Plasma progesterone

1. male < 2 nmol/l
2. female (follicular phase) 0–2 nmol/l
3. female (luteal phase) > 20 nmol/l

Plasma testosterone

1. male 11–36 nmol/l
2. female 0·7–2·5 nmol/l

Pancreas

Plasma glucose
Fasting level $< 6·5$ mmol/l
2 h post prandial $< 7·0$ mmol/l
Hypoglycaemic levels < 2 mmol/l

Parathyroid

Serum calcium 2·2–2·6 mmol/l
Serum inorganic phosphorus 0·8–1·5 mmol/l
Serum alkaline phosphatase 80–280 U/l
Plasma parathormone 200–600 ng/l

Pituitary

1. Hypothalamic-pituitary adrenal axis: normal response to hypoglycaemia is plasma 'cortisol' increment > 200 nmol/l with final value > 550 nmol/l
Plasma ACTH 0–80 ng/l

2. TRH test—see thyroid tests
3. Gonadotrophin levels
   FSH male 3–8 U/1
   female 3–10 U/1
   LH male 3–10 U/1
   female 3–15 U/1
   GnRH test: normal response is increment of serum FSH > 2 U/1 and increment of serum LH of 3–20 U/1
4. Growth Hormone value during hypoglycaemia > 20μU/ml

Index

CHURCHILL LIVINGSTONE MEDICAL TEXTS

Epidemiology in Medical Practice
Second edition
D. J. P. Barker and C. Rose

Pain: its Nature, Analysis and Treatment
Michael R. Bond

Essentials of Dermatology
J. L. Burton

An Introduction to Clinical Rheumatology
Second edition
William Carson Dick

Elements of Medical Genetics
Fifth edition
Alan E. H. Emery

Notes on Psychiatry
Fifth edition
I. M. Ingram, G. C. Timbury and R. M. Mowbray

Physiology: a Clinical Approach
Third edition
G. R. Kelman

A Concise Textbook of Gastroenterology
Second edition
M. J. S. Langman

Tumours: Basic Principles and Clinical Aspects
Christopher Louis

Nutrition and its Disorders
Third edition
Donald S. McLaren

The Essentials of Neuroanatomy
Third edition
G. A. G. Mitchell and D. Mayor

Clinical Bacteriology
P. W. Ross

Sexually Transmitted Diseases
Third edition
C. B. S. Schofield

Respiratory Medicine
Second edition
Malcolm Schonell

An Introduction to General Pathology
Second edition
W. G. Spector

Child Psychiatry for Students
Second edition
Frederick H. Stone and Cyrille Koupernik

Notes on Medical Virology
Sixth edition
Morag C. Timbury

Clinical Pharmacology
Third edition
P. Turner and A. Richens

Immunology: an Outline for Students of Medicine and Biology
Fourth edition
D. M. Weir

Clinical Thinking and Practice: Diagnosis and Decision in Patient Care
H. J. Wright and D. B. MacAdam

LIVINGSTONE MEDICAL TEXTS

Geriatric Medicine for Students
J. C. Brocklehurst and T. Hanley

Introduction to Clinical Examination
Second edition
Edited by John Macleod

An Introduction to Primary Medical Care
David Morrell

Urology and Renal Medicine
Second edition
J. B. Newman and J. J. B. Petrie

Psychological Medicine for Students
John Pollitt

Cardiology for Students
Max Zoob